W0106477

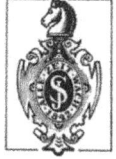

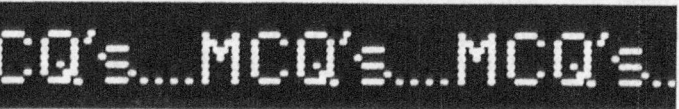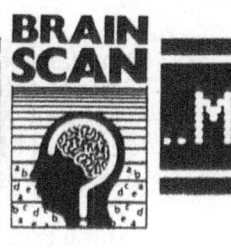

Norman Johnson · Anton Pozniak

MRCP Part I

Springer-Verlag
Berlin Heidelberg New York
London Paris Tokyo

Norman Johnson, MD, MRCP
Senior Lecturer in Medicine and Honorary Consultant
Physician, Middlesex and University College Hospitals
School of Medicine, The Middlesex Hospital, Mortimer
Street, London W1N 8AA, England

Anton Pozniak, MB, ChB, MRCP
Formerly Registrar, Department of Medicine,
The Middlesex Hospital Medical School, Mortimer Street,
London W1N 8AA, England

Publisher's note: the 'Brainscan' logo is reproduced by courtesy of The
Editor, Geriatric Medicine, Modern Medicine GB Ltd.

ISBN-13: 978-3-540-16215-5   e-ISBN-13: 978-1-4471-1413-0
DOI: 10.1007/978-1-4471-1413-0

This work is subject to copyright. All rights reserved, whether the whole or
part of the material is concerned, specifically those of translation, reprinting,
re-use of illustrations, broadcasting, reproduction by photocopying,
machine or similar means, and storage in data banks.

© Springer-Verlag Berlin Heidelberg 1986

The use of registered names, trademarks, etc, in this publication does not
imply, even in the absence of a specific statement, that such names are
exempt from the relevant protective laws and regulations and therefore free
for general use.

Filmset by Wilmaset, Birkenhead, Wirral
Printed by Page Bros (Norwich) Ltd, Mile Cross Lane, Norwich

2128/3916–543210

Contents

Introduction to MRCP Part I

Multiple choice questions have been a popular way of setting exams for at least 20 years. However fair or unfair they appear to be, they are destined to remain a part of the system. The main reason for their popularity is that they provide a compact method of testing the candidate's knowledge over a very wide field. This is an obvious advantage in a subject such as Medicine. Multiple choice questions allow easy and unbiased marking which can be performed rapidly by computer. Computerised marking also facilitates qualitative control of questions and statistical analysis of the exam. In order to discourage wild guessing a heavy penalty is introduced in the form of a negative score for an incorrect answer which usually results in candidates' answer sheets being returned with a proportion of 'don't knows'.

The MRCP Part I examination is held three times a year in many centres in the United Kingdom and abroad. A maximum of four attempts at Part I are allowed. Re-entry may be deferred if the candidate fails badly. No set syllabus is published by the Royal Colleges but recently the emphasis of the exam has been on the basic sciences, which will comprise up to 30% of the exam. Sixty multiple choice questions are used from an ever-changing bank of about 4000 questions. A breakdown of the relative distribution of questions is given below.

Topic	No. of questions asked
Anatomy	1
Cardiology	4
Clinical pharmacology	5
Dermatology	1
Endocrinology	3
Gastroenterology	1
Genetics	1
Haematology	2 or 3
Immunology or allergy	1

Industrial medicine	1
Infectious diseases	2 or 3
Metabolic disease	2
Musculoskeletal diseases	2
Neurology	4
Ophthalmology	1
Paediatrics	4
Physiology	1
Psychiatry	4
Renal disease	3
Respiratory diseases	4
Reticuloendothelial system	1
Statistics	1
Symptoms and signs	1 or 2
Toxicology	1
Tropical medicine	1 or 0

The exam is essentially competitive, with about the top 30% of candidates passing each time, the passmark therefore being variable. In simple terms, this means that the successful candidate must perform better than the majority of his or her colleagues. Achieving this requires sound knowledge of medicine and basic science, as well as practice in multiple choice question technique.

There is no doubt that at least 12 weeks' serious preparatory work is needed for this exam. A busy clinical job can erode the time spent in the proper preparation which is so necessary for success.

Stage I: This should be a stage of broadly based general reading (see list below), aimed at acquiring good background knowledge.

Stage II: This should be one of using subject-based multiple choice questions to guide detailed reading in areas of weakness. This helps to highlight the fields in which additional reading is valuable. Using multiple choice questions in this way helps the candidate to be guided into those areas on which the College has placed particular emphasis.

Stage III: This stage of preparation for the exam is the most difficult. Many candidates find it hard to take an overall view, but working through multiple choice question papers is probably the best way to polish technique and pick out any final points requiring extra attention. This method also enables one to gain insight into one's own aptitude for multiple choice question exams, which is invaluable when actually sitting the paper. The College quite rightly advise against guessing, but one only learns to assess reasonable certainty by practice and experience.

Bibliography

Bannister R (1985) Brain's clinical neurology, 6th edn. Oxford University Press, London

Burton JL (1983) Aids to postgraduate medicine, 4th edn. Churchill Livingstone, London

Crofton J, Douglas A (1981) Respiratory diseases, 3rd edn. Blackwell, Oxford

Davies IJT (1983) Postgraduate medicine, 4th edn. Lloyd-Luke, London

Dixon MF (1986) Aids to pathology, 3rd edn. Churchill Livingstone, London

Eastham RD (1985) Biochemical values in clinical medicine, 7th edn. John Wright, Bristol

Forfar JO, Arneil GC (1984) Textbook of paediatrics, vols 1 and 2, 3rd edn. Churchill Livingstone, London

Gabriel R (1985) Postgraduate nephrology, 3rd edn. Butterworth, London

Gabriel R, Gabriel CM (1983) Medical lists for examinations. Butterworth, London

Ganong WF (1985) Review of medical physiology, 12th edn. Lange, California

Goodman LS, Gilman A (1985) The pharmacological basis of therapeutics, 7th edn. MacMillan, New York

Huskisson EC, Dudley Hart F (1978) All the arthropathies, 3rd edn. John Wright, Bristol

Isselbacher KJ et al. (eds) (1983) Harrison's principles of internal medicine. McGraw Hill, New York

Johnson NMcI (1986) Respiratory medicine. Blackwell Scientific, Oxford

Laurence DR, Bennett PN (1980) Clinical pharmacology, 5th edn. Churchill Livingstone, London

Rogers H, Spector R (1984) Aids to clinical pharmacology with therapeutics. Churchill Livingstone, London

Roitt I (1984) Essential immunology, 5th edn. Blackwell, London

Rubenstein D, Wayne D (1985) Lecture notes on clinical medicine, 3rd edn. Blackwell Scientific, London

Schamroth L (1982) An introduction to electrocardiography, 6th edn. Blackwell Scientific, London

Sherlock S (1985) Disease of the liver and biliary system, 7th edn. Blackwell, London

Snell RS (1981) Clinical anatomy for medical students, 2nd edn. Little, Brown & Co, Boston

Weatherall DJ, Leadingham JGG, Warrell DA (1983) The

Oxford textbook of medicine, 1st edn. Oxford University Press, London
Zilva JF, Pannall P (1984) Clinical chemistry in diagnosis and treatment, 4th edn. Churchill Livingstone, London

Examples of Multiple Choice Questions from the Common Part I MRCP (UK), 1st and 2nd series. Royal College of Physicians of Edinburgh, Glasgow and London
Medicine International vols 1 and 2, 1982 onwards. Oxford

Journals: British Medical Journal
British Journal of Hospital Medicine
Hospital Update
The Lancet
New England Journal of Medicine

Addresses of Royal Colleges

Royal College of Physicians of Edinburgh
9 Queen Street
Edinburgh EH2 1JQ

Royal College of Physicians of Glasgow
242 St Vincent Street
Glasgow G2 5RJ

Royal College of Physicians of London
11 St Andrews Place
Regents Park
London NW1 4LE

How to Use this Book

All of these examination papers have been used in the Bloomsbury MRCP Part I Course which we organise. The passmark given for each paper (with each answer sheet) gives a guide to the performance of previous candidates who have been successful in the membership.

You should use this book as a set of test examinations to be taken in stage III of your revision. By doing so, not only will you gain experience of performing under the stress of a time limit, but you will also be able to assess your strengths and weaknesses. Don't forget to read the questions carefully, check your answers and fill in the answer sheet correctly.

The Examination

1. You are allowed 2 hours to complete the paper, which is answered on a computer card (see below) with a 2B pencil.

2. Each initial statement or stem has five possible completions, listed A, B, C, D and E.

3. Each of these has to be answered 'true', 'false' or 'don't know' by filling in the appropriate box on the answer sheet.

4. There is no restriction on the number of true or false answers to any question.

Examination 1

All parts of every Question must be answered *True* or *False* or *Don't Know* by filling in the box provided. Failure to do so will result in rejection of the answer sheet

✂

EXAMINATION NO.
1

SURNAME

INITIALS

Please use 2B PENCIL only. Rub out all errors thoroughly.
Mark lozenges like ▬ NOT like this ⊘ ⊘ ⊗

T ⊂⊃ = TRUE   F ⊂⊃ = FALSE   DK ⊂⊃ = DON'T KNOW

	A	B	C	D	E		A	B	C	D	E
1	T / F / DK	T / F / DK	T / F / DK	T / F / DK	T / F / DK	16	T / F / DK	T / F / DK	T / F / DK	T / F / DK	T / F / DK
2	T / F / DK	T / F / DK	T / F / DK	T / F / DK	T / F / DK	17	T / F / DK	T / F / DK	T / F / DK	T / F / DK	T / F / DK
3	T / F / DK	T / F / DK	T / F / DK	T / F / DK	T / F / DK	18	T / F / DK	T / F / DK	T / F / DK	T / F / DK	T / F / DK
4	T / F / DK	T / F / DK	T / F / DK	T / F / DK	T / F / DK	19	T / F / DK	T / F / DK	T / F / DK	T / F / DK	T / F / DK
5	T / F / DK	T / F / DK	T / F / DK	T / F / DK	T / F / DK	20	T / F / DK	T / F / DK	T / F / DK	T / F / DK	T / F / DK
6	T / F / DK	T / F / DK	T / F / DK	T / F / DK	T / F / DK	21	T / F / DK	T / F / DK	T / F / DK	T / F / DK	T / F / DK
7	T / F / DK	T / F / DK	T / F / DK	T / F / DK	T / F / DK	22	T / F / DK	T / F / DK	T / F / DK	T / F / DK	T / F / DK
8	T / F / DK	T / F / DK	T / F / DK	T / F / DK	T / F / DK	23	T / F / DK	T / F / DK	T / F / DK	T / F / DK	T / F / DK
9	T / F / DK	T / F / DK	T / F / DK	T / F / DK	T / F / DK	24	T / F / DK	T / F / DK	T / F / DK	T / F / DK	T / F / DK
10	T / F / DK	T / F / DK	T / F / DK	T / F / DK	T / F / DK	25	T / F / DK	T / F / DK	T / F / DK	T / F / DK	T / F / DK
11	T / F / DK	T / F / DK	T / F / DK	T / F / DK	T / F / DK	26	T / F / DK	T / F / DK	T / F / DK	T / F / DK	T / F / DK
12	T / F / DK	T / F / DK	T / F / DK	T / F / DK	T / F / DK	27	T / F / DK	T / F / DK	T / F / DK	T / F / DK	T / F / DK
13	T / F / DK	T / F / DK	T / F / DK	T / F / DK	T / F / DK	28	T / F / DK	T / F / DK	T / F / DK	T / F / DK	T / F / DK
14	T / F / DK	T / F / DK	T / F / DK	T / F / DK	T / F / DK	29	T / F / DK	T / F / DK	T / F / DK	T / F / DK	T / F / DK
15	T / F / DK	T / F / DK	T / F / DK	T / F / DK	T / F / DK	30	T / F / DK	T / F / DK	T / F / DK	T / F / DK	T / F / DK

	A	B	C	D	E
31	T ☐ / F ☐ / DK ☐	T ☐ / F ☐ / DK ☐	T ☐ / F ☐ / DK ☐	T ☐ / F ☐ / DK ☐	T ☐ / F ☐ / DK ☐
32	T ☐ / F ☐ / DK ☐	T ☐ / F ☐ / DK ☐	T ☐ / F ☐ / DK ☐	T ☐ / F ☐ / DK ☐	T ☐ / F ☐ / DK ☐
33	T ☐ / F ☐ / DK ☐	T ☐ / F ☐ / DK ☐	T ☐ / F ☐ / DK ☐	T ☐ / F ☐ / DK ☐	T ☐ / F ☐ / DK ☐
34	T ☐ / F ☐ / DK ☐	T ☐ / F ☐ / DK ☐	T ☐ / F ☐ / DK ☐	T ☐ / F ☐ / DK ☐	T ☐ / F ☐ / DK ☐
35	T ☐ / F ☐ / DK ☐	T ☐ / F ☐ / DK ☐	T ☐ / F ☐ / DK ☐	T ☐ / F ☐ / DK ☐	T ☐ / F ☐ / DK ☐
36	T ☐ / F ☐ / DK ☐	T ☐ / F ☐ / DK ☐	T ☐ / F ☐ / DK ☐	T ☐ / F ☐ / DK ☐	T ☐ / F ☐ / DK ☐
37	T ☐ / F ☐ / DK ☐	T ☐ / F ☐ / DK ☐	T ☐ / F ☐ / DK ☐	T ☐ / F ☐ / DK ☐	T ☐ / F ☐ / DK ☐
38	T ☐ / F ☐ / DK ☐	T ☐ / F ☐ / DK ☐	T ☐ / F ☐ / DK ☐	T ☐ / F ☐ / DK ☐	T ☐ / F ☐ / DK ☐
39	T ☐ / F ☐ / DK ☐	T ☐ / F ☐ / DK ☐	T ☐ / F ☐ / DK ☐	T ☐ / F ☐ / DK ☐	T ☐ / F ☐ / DK ☐
40	T ☐ / F ☐ / DK ☐	T ☐ / F ☐ / DK ☐	T ☐ / F ☐ / DK ☐	T ☐ / F ☐ / DK ☐	T ☐ / F ☐ / DK ☐
41	T ☐ / F ☐ / DK ☐	T ☐ / F ☐ / DK ☐	T ☐ / F ☐ / DK ☐	T ☐ / F ☐ / DK ☐	T ☐ / F ☐ / DK ☐
42	T ☐ / F ☐ / DK ☐	T ☐ / F ☐ / DK ☐	T ☐ / F ☐ / DK ☐	T ☐ / F ☐ / DK ☐	T ☐ / F ☐ / DK ☐
43	T ☐ / F ☐ / DK ☐	T ☐ / F ☐ / DK ☐	T ☐ / F ☐ / DK ☐	T ☐ / F ☐ / DK ☐	T ☐ / F ☐ / DK ☐
44	T ☐ / F ☐ / DK ☐	T ☐ / F ☐ / DK ☐	T ☐ / F ☐ / DK ☐	T ☐ / F ☐ / DK ☐	T ☐ / F ☐ / DK ☐
45	T ☐ / F ☐ / DK ☐	T ☐ / F ☐ / DK ☐	T ☐ / F ☐ / DK ☐	T ☐ / F ☐ / DK ☐	T ☐ / F ☐ / DK ☐

	A	B	C	D	E
46	T ☐ / F ☐ / DK ☐	T ☐ / F ☐ / DK ☐	T ☐ / F ☐ / DK ☐	T ☐ / F ☐ / DK ☐	T ☐ / F ☐ / DK ☐
47	T ☐ / F ☐ / DK ☐	T ☐ / F ☐ / DK ☐	T ☐ / F ☐ / DK ☐	T ☐ / F ☐ / DK ☐	T ☐ / F ☐ / DK ☐
48	T ☐ / F ☐ / DK ☐	T ☐ / F ☐ / DK ☐	T ☐ / F ☐ / DK ☐	T ☐ / F ☐ / DK ☐	T ☐ / F ☐ / DK ☐
49	T ☐ / F ☐ / DK ☐	T ☐ / F ☐ / DK ☐	T ☐ / F ☐ / DK ☐	T ☐ / F ☐ / DK ☐	T ☐ / F ☐ / DK ☐
50	T ☐ / F ☐ / DK ☐	T ☐ / F ☐ / DK ☐	T ☐ / F ☐ / DK ☐	T ☐ / F ☐ / DK ☐	T ☐ / F ☐ / DK ☐
51	T ☐ / F ☐ / DK ☐	T ☐ / F ☐ / DK ☐	T ☐ / F ☐ / DK ☐	T ☐ / F ☐ / DK ☐	T ☐ / F ☐ / DK ☐
52	T ☐ / F ☐ / DK ☐	T ☐ / F ☐ / DK ☐	T ☐ / F ☐ / DK ☐	T ☐ / F ☐ / DK ☐	T ☐ / F ☐ / DK ☐
53	T ☐ / F ☐ / DK ☐	T ☐ / F ☐ / DK ☐	T ☐ / F ☐ / DK ☐	T ☐ / F ☐ / DK ☐	T ☐ / F ☐ / DK ☐
54	T ☐ / F ☐ / DK ☐	T ☐ / F ☐ / DK ☐	T ☐ / F ☐ / DK ☐	T ☐ / F ☐ / DK ☐	T ☐ / F ☐ / DK ☐
55	T ☐ / F ☐ / DK ☐	T ☐ / F ☐ / DK ☐	T ☐ / F ☐ / DK ☐	T ☐ / F ☐ / DK ☐	T ☐ / F ☐ / DK ☐
56	T ☐ / F ☐ / DK ☐	T ☐ / F ☐ / DK ☐	T ☐ / F ☐ / DK ☐	T ☐ / F ☐ / DK ☐	T ☐ / F ☐ / DK ☐
57	T ☐ / F ☐ / DK ☐	T ☐ / F ☐ / DK ☐	T ☐ / F ☐ / DK ☐	T ☐ / F ☐ / DK ☐	T ☐ / F ☐ / DK ☐
58	T ☐ / F ☐ / DK ☐	T ☐ / F ☐ / DK ☐	T ☐ / F ☐ / DK ☐	T ☐ / F ☐ / DK ☐	T ☐ / F ☐ / DK ☐
59	T ☐ / F ☐ / DK ☐	T ☐ / F ☐ / DK ☐	T ☐ / F ☐ / DK ☐	T ☐ / F ☐ / DK ☐	T ☐ / F ☐ / DK ☐
60	T ☐ / F ☐ / DK ☐	T ☐ / F ☐ / DK ☐	T ☐ / F ☐ / DK ☐	T ☐ / F ☐ / DK ☐	T ☐ / F ☐ / DK ☐

1. Which of the following statements concerning depression are true?

   a) Illusionary misinterpretation is common
   b) Physical symptoms are common
   c) Muscle tone is increased
   d) Retardation occurs
   e) Gustatory hallucinations occur

2. Petit mal:

   a) Often presents in the 3rd decade
   b) Is associated with narcolepsy
   c) Should be treated with phenytoin
   d) May present with learning problems
   e) Usually proceeds to grand mal fits

3. Parkinsonism may result from:

   a) Lead poisoning
   b) Wilson's disease
   c) Mercury poisoning
   d) Carbon dioxide retention
   e) Kernicterus

4. Which of the following are inherited in an autosomal recessive manner?

   a) Hereditary spherocytosis
   b) Christmas disease
   c) Glucose-6-phosphate dehydrogenase deficiency
   d) Von Willebrand's disease
   e) Achondroplasia

5. Which of the following may be caused by paracetamol overdose?

   a) Hyperglycaemia
   b) Renal tubular necrosis
   c) Encephalopathy
   d) Phasic nystagmus
   e) Sagittal sinus thrombosis

6. Which helminth is paired with the anti-helminthic of choice?

a) Fascioliasis — niridazole
b) Onchocerciasis — suramin
c) Schistosomiasis — niclosamide
d) *Taenia saginata* — antimony salts
e) Paragonimiasis — bithionol

7. In measles:

a) The incubation period is 1 week
b) Splenomegaly is common
c) Photophobia is frequent
d) Koplik spots are common (>50%)
e) Lymphadenopathy is marked

8. Respiratory syncytial virus infection:

a) Causes bronchiolitis
b) Causes a maculopapular rash
c) May be prevented by vaccination
d) Causes a leucocytosis
e) Causes severe pharyngitis

9. Which of the following are associated with mental retardation?

a) Cystinuria
b) Niemann-Pick's disease
c) Achondroplasia
d) Galactosaemia
e) Muscular dystrophy

10. In Korsakoff's psychosis:

a) Treatment with thiamine is curative
b) Red cell transketolase is raised
c) Anterograde amnesia occurs
d) Depression is a major feature
e) Confabulation is characteristic

11. Which of the following are true?

   a) The standard deviation (SD) is greater than the standard error of the mean (SEM)
   b) The SEM determines the accuracy of measurement of the observations
   c) The SD is a measure of observation variability
   d) $SD = SEM/\sqrt{n}$
   e) The SD equals the SEM in non-parametric tests

12. The normal metabolic response to major surgery includes:

   a) Natriuresis
   b) Glycogenolysis
   c) Antidiuresis
   d) Negative nitrogen balance
   e) Increased tidal volume

13. Which are true of therapy in oat cell carcinoma of the bronchus?

   a) Surgery is of less benefit than with squamous cell cancer
   b) Chemotherapy causes 50% complete remission in limited disease
   c) CNS irradiation may lead to memory loss
   d) Radiotherapy is a useful adjuvant to chemotherapy
   e) Prognosis with limited disease given chemotherapy is 3 months

14. Periodic breathing occurs in:

   a) Cerebral contusion
   b) Deep sea diving bells
   c) Uraemia
   d) Normals
   e) Myxoedema

15. Which of the following may cause sleep apnoea?

   a) Alzheimer's disease
   b) Hypokalaemia
   c) Acromegaly
   d) Obesity
   e) Tetanus

16. Renal blood flow:

    a) Is 40% of the cardiac output at rest
    b) Can be measured using the Fick principle
    c) Is higher in the medulla than the cortex
    d) Is increased when renal nerves are stimulated
    e) Is decreased in response to hypoxia

17. In cystic fibrosis:

    a) 1:2000 of all births are affected
    b) Meconium ileus is a common presenting feature
    c) All newborn infants are now screened in the UK
    d) Immunisation against measles is contraindicated
    e) Diabetes mellitus may occur in adolescence

18. Which of the following may cause mediastinal
    lymphadenopathy?

    a) Phenytoin
    b) AIDS
    c) Carcinoma of the bronchus
    d) Thymoma
    e) Carcinoma of the breast

19. Renal calculi may be caused by:

    a) Medullary sponge kidney
    b) Hypoparathyroidism
    c) Hypercalciuria
    d) Renal tubular acidosis
    e) Primary hyperparathyroidism

20. Which of these renal stones are radio–opaque?

    a) Cystine
    b) Xanthine
    c) Uric acid
    d) Oxalate
    e) Silicate

21. Which of these statements concerning Down's syndrome are true?

   a) Translocation of chromosomes is the commonest cause
   b) A Simian crease is diagnostic
   c) Abnormal dermatoglyphics are usual
   d) The occiput is prominent
   e) A "floppy" baby may be the presenting feature

22. In children, haematuria:

   a) Is usually due to an underlying serious condition
   b) May be due to infection with adenovirus II
   c) May be associated with nerve deafness
   d) Is benign in Henoch-Schönlein purpura
   e) Should be investigated by cystoscopy in most cases

23. Marasmus:

   a) Is commoner in twins
   b) Is due to protein deficiency
   c) May be associated with severe chronic bowel disease
   d) The risk of superadded infection is high during recovery
   e) The recovery of older children is much greater than younger

24. Cyanosis is usual at birth in:

   a) Fallot's tetralogy
   b) Transposition of the great arteries
   c) Maladie de Roger
   d) Pulmonary stenosis
   e) Hypoplastic left heart

25. Lithium toxicity may present with:

   a) Hypertension
   b) Jaundice
   c) Apathy
   d) Haemorrhage
   e) Convulsions

26. Which of the following may follow a myocardial infarction?
    a) Ruptured cordae leading to tricuspid incompetence
    b) Cannon waves
    c) Pericarditis
    d) Cerebral embolisation
    e) Raised γ-glutamyl transferase

27. Which of the following drugs in their usual dose may cause toxicity in patients with renal failure?
    a) Phenytoin
    b) Chlorpropramide
    c) Tolbutamide
    d) Neomycin
    e) Digitoxin

28. Jaundice may result from therapy with:
    a) Isoniazid
    b) Rifampicin
    c) Pyrazinamide
    d) Cycloserine
    e) Capreomycin

29. Which of the following are useful in the therapy of Raynaud's phenomenon?
    a) Prostacyclin
    b) Alcohol
    c) Terfenadine
    d) Nifedipine
    e) Propantheline

30. Which of these drugs have ocular complications?
    a) Pyrimethamine
    b) Atenolol
    c) Methotrexate
    d) Chloroquine
    e) Ethambutol

31. 1,25$(OH)_2D_3$ (1,25 vitamin D):

   a) Stimulates the absorption of calcium and phosphate from the gut
   b) Stimulates calcium and phosphate resorption from bone
   c) Stimulates the excretion of calcium and phosphate into renal tubules
   d) Levels are low during lactation
   e) Is more active a metabolite than 24,25-OH_2 vitamin D

32. Which of the following are true?

   a) Osmolality is the number of osmoles of solute per kilogram of solvent
   b) Osmolality can be calculated from 2(Na^+ + K^+) + glucose + chloride mmol/litre
   c) In ethanol poisoning, the measured osmolality can exceed calculated osmolality
   d) One osmole of a substance depresses the freezing point of a solvent by 1.86°C
   e) The main determinant of intracellular fluid osmolality is intracellular potassium concentration

33. The vagus:

   a) Supplies the larynx
   b) Bronchodilates
   c) Speeds the heart
   d) Stimulates gastric acid secretion
   e) Innervates the diaphragm

34. Which of the following are lymphokines?

   a) IgM
   b) Eosinophil chemotactic factor
   c) γ-Interferon
   d) C1q
   e) Secretory piece

35. Which of these statements concerning Reiter's disease are true?

   a) The knee is most commonly affected
   b) May follow *Campylobacter* infection
   c) Is associated with an increased incidence of venous thrombosis
   d) Rarely recurs
   e) Anterior uveitis is an early manifestation

36. Worsening of SLE may be due to:

   a) Pregnancy
   b) Hydralazine therapy
   c) Winter holiday in Lapland
   d) Procainamide therapy
   e) Salbutamol therapy

37. In rheumatoid arthritis:

   a) Nodules commonly occur in seronegative rheumatoid disease
   b) *Staphylococcus aureus* is the commonest infection in joints
   c) Proximal ulnar erosions are common
   d) Subchondrial cysts are common
   e) Finger drop is commoner in young females

38. Optic atrophy may occur in:

   a) Tobacco amblyopia
   b) Amaurosis fugax
   c) Carbon tetrachloride poisoning
   d) Disseminated sclerosis
   e) Papilloedema

39. A giant spleen may result from:

   a) Glandular fever
   b) Secondary polycythaemia
   c) Typhoid
   d) Myelofibrosis
   e) Sarcoidosis

40. Which of the following may be associated with ulcerative colitis?

   a) Ascending cholangitis
   b) Cholangiocarcinoma
   c) Chronic active hepatitis
   d) Cirrhosis
   e) Cholelithiasis

41. In ascites which are true?

   a) There is a low protein content in right heart failure
   b) There are numerous acid fast bacilli if tuberculosis is the
      cause
   c) Ovarian carcinoma is a rare cause in women
   d) Atypical lymphocytes in the fluid suggest glandular fever
   e) There is a high angiotensin converting enzyme level with a
      malignant cause

42. H_2 antagonists:

   a) Speed gastric emptying
   b) Cause bronchodilation
   c) Increase pancreatic secretion
   d) Increase gastric pH
   e) Improve symptoms of hiatus hernia

43. Ring lesions on the skin may be due to:

   a) Pityriasis rosea
   b) Pityriasis versicolor
   c) Lichen planus
   d) Granuloma annulare
   e) Erythema induratum

44. Sideroblastic anaemia:

   a) Is characterised by intracellular iron-laden mitochondria
   b) Is caused by antituberculous drugs
   c) Is caused by pyridoxine deficiency
   d) Is associated with a low neutrophil alkaline phosphatase
      score
   e) Is characterised by anti-I antibodies on red blood cells

45. Which of the following are converted to an active metabolite?

   a) Morphine
   b) Nortriptyline
   c) Amitriptyline
   d) Cyclophosphamide
   e) Phenacetin

46. Acute iritis can be secondary to:

a) Keratoconus
b) Psoriasis
c) Reiter's syndrome
d) Lyme arthritis
e) Osteogenesis imperfecta

47. Sudden blindness may result from:

a) Diabetes mellitus
b) Migraine
c) Epilepsy
d) Retinal vein thrombosis
e) Meningioma

48. Heinz bodies may result from:

a) Sickle cell anaemia
b) Glucose-6-phosphate dehydrogenase deficiency
c) Favism
d) Thalassaemia
e) Drug-induced haemolysis

49. Causes of osteoporosis include:

a) Thyrotoxicosis
b) Alcoholism
c) Addison's disease
d) Space travel
e) Sarcoidosis

50. Glucocorticoid therapy may cause:

a) Hypokalaemia
b) Lymphopenia
c) Hypertrichosis
d) Amenorrhoea
e) Aseptic necrosis of the femoral head

51. Hypoglycaemia may occur in association with:

a) Elevated C peptide levels
b) Liver failure
c) Diabetes insipidus
d) Fibrosarcoma
e) Untreated diabetes mellitus

52. Maculopapular rashes occur with:

a) Typhoid
b) Syphilis
c) Anthrax
d) Rubella
e) Hand, foot and mouth disease

53. Cardiomyopathy may result from:

a) Haemochromatosis
b) Sarcoidosis
c) Toxoplasmosis
d) Freidreich's ataxia
e) Cobalt poisoning

54. Cavitating pneumonia is characteristically caused by which of the following?

a) Histoplasmosis
b) *Micropolysporum faenii*
c) *Legionella pneumophila*
d) *Mycoplasma pneumonia*
e) Klebsiella spp.

55. Concerning the membrane potential of cardiac muscle:

a) Phase 0 shows a slow and steady rise in potential
b) Phase 2 is associated with efflux of calcium ions
c) Phase 3 is produced by an efflux of potassium ions
d) Slowing of phase 3 decreases the QT interval
e) Verapamil blocks slow calcium currents

56. Loudness of the first heart sounds occurs in:

a) Mitral reflux
b) First degree heart block
c) Wolff-Parkinson-White syndrome
d) Atrial flutter
e) Atrial septal defect

57. Cyanosis may be caused by:

a) A P_aO_2 of 80 mmHg in a patient with polycythaemia
b) Eisenmenger's syndrome
c) Carbon monoxide poisoning
d) The bends
e) 5 g% reduced Hb

58. Gastrin:

a) Is secreted by antral cells
b) Is secreted by duodenal cells
c) May be inactivated in the kidney
d) Stimulates the growth of gastric mucosa
e) Stimulates insulin after a carbohydrate meal

59. Which of the following are true?

a) C_1 esterase levels are low in angioedema
b) Immune complex levels are elevated in active tuberculosis
c) The phytohaemagglutinin response is increased in Hodgkin's disease
d) CH_{50} is low in SLE
e) There is a polyclonal increase in immunoglobulins in sarcoidosis

60. Which of the following organisms commonly cause pneumonia in AIDS?

a) Cytomegalovirus
b) *Mycobacterium avium-intracellulare*
c) *Mycobacterium tuberculosis*
d) *Pneumocystis carinii*
e) Herpes simplex

Examination 2

All parts of every Question must be answered *True* or *False* or *Don't Know* by filling in the box provided. Failure to do so will result in rejection of the answer sheet

✂

EXAMINATION NO.

2

SURNAME

| | | | | | | | | | | | | | | | | | | | | | |

INITIALS

| | | | |

Please use 2B PENCIL only. Rub out all errors thoroughly.
Mark lozenges like ▬ NOT like this ⌀ ⌀ ⌀

T ⊂⊃ = TRUE   F ⊂⊃ = FALSE   DK ⊂⊃ = DON'T KNOW

	A	B	C	D	E		A	B	C	D	E
1	T / F / DK	T / F / DK	T / F / DK	T / F / DK	T / F / DK	16	T / F / DK	T / F / DK	T / F / DK	T / F / DK	T / F / DK
2	T / F / DK	T / F / DK	T / F / DK	T / F / DK	T / F / DK	17	T / F / DK	T / F / DK	T / F / DK	T / F / DK	T / F / DK
3	T / F / DK	T / F / DK	T / F / DK	T / F / DK	T / F / DK	18	T / F / DK	T / F / DK	T / F / DK	T / F / DK	T / F / DK
4	T / F / DK	T / F / DK	T / F / DK	T / F / DK	T / F / DK	19	T / F / DK	T / F / DK	T / F / DK	T / F / DK	T / F / DK
5	T / F / DK	T / F / DK	T / F / DK	T / F / DK	T / F / DK	20	T / F / DK	T / F / DK	T / F / DK	T / F / DK	T / F / DK
6	T / F / DK	T / F / DK	T / F / DK	T / F / DK	T / F / DK	21	T / F / DK	T / F / DK	T / F / DK	T / F / DK	T / F / DK
7	T / F / DK	T / F / DK	T / F / DK	T / F / DK	T / F / DK	22	T / F / DK	T / F / DK	T / F / DK	T / F / DK	T / F / DK
8	T / F / DK	T / F / DK	T / F / DK	T / F / DK	T / F / DK	23	T / F / DK	T / F / DK	T / F / DK	T / F / DK	T / F / DK
9	T / F / DK	T / F / DK	T / F / DK	T / F / DK	T / F / DK	24	T / F / DK	T / F / DK	T / F / DK	T / F / DK	T / F / DK
10	T / F / DK	T / F / DK	T / F / DK	T / F / DK	T / F / DK	25	T / F / DK	T / F / DK	T / F / DK	T / F / DK	T / F / DK
11	T / F / DK	T / F / DK	T / F / DK	T / F / DK	T / F / DK	26	T / F / DK	T / F / DK	T / F / DK	T / F / DK	T / F / DK
12	T / F / DK	T / F / DK	T / F / DK	T / F / DK	T / F / DK	27	T / F / DK	T / F / DK	T / F / DK	T / F / DK	T / F / DK
13	T / F / DK	T / F / DK	T / F / DK	T / F / DK	T / F / DK	28	T / F / DK	T / F / DK	T / F / DK	T / F / DK	T / F / DK
14	T / F / DK	T / F / DK	T / F / DK	T / F / DK	T / F / DK	29	T / F / DK	T / F / DK	T / F / DK	T / F / DK	T / F / DK
15	T / F / DK	T / F / DK	T / F / DK	T / F / DK	T / F / DK	30	T / F / DK	T / F / DK	T / F / DK	T / F / DK	T / F / DK

	A	B	C	D	E		A	B	C	D	E
31	T ◯ F ◯ DK ◯	T ◯ F ◯ DK ◯	T ◯ F ◯ DK ◯	T ◯ F ◯ DK ◯	T ◯ F ◯ DK ◯	**46**	T ◯ F ◯ DK ◯	T ◯ F ◯ DK ◯	T ◯ F ◯ DK ◯	T ◯ F ◯ DK ◯	T ◯ F ◯ DK ◯
32	T ◯ F ◯ DK ◯	T ◯ F ◯ DK ◯	T ◯ F ◯ DK ◯	T ◯ F ◯ DK ◯	T ◯ F ◯ DK ◯	**47**	T ◯ F ◯ DK ◯	T ◯ F ◯ DK ◯	T ◯ F ◯ DK ◯	T ◯ F ◯ DK ◯	T ◯ F ◯ DK ◯
33	T ◯ F ◯ DK ◯	T ◯ F ◯ DK ◯	T ◯ F ◯ DK ◯	T ◯ F ◯ DK ◯	T ◯ F ◯ DK ◯	**48**	T ◯ F ◯ DK ◯	T ◯ F ◯ DK ◯	T ◯ F ◯ DK ◯	T ◯ F ◯ DK ◯	T ◯ F ◯ DK ◯
34	T ◯ F ◯ DK ◯	T ◯ F ◯ DK ◯	T ◯ F ◯ DK ◯	T ◯ F ◯ DK ◯	T ◯ F ◯ DK ◯	**49**	T ◯ F ◯ DK ◯	T ◯ F ◯ DK ◯	T ◯ F ◯ DK ◯	T ◯ F ◯ DK ◯	T ◯ F ◯ DK ◯
35	T ◯ F ◯ DK ◯	T ◯ F ◯ DK ◯	T ◯ F ◯ DK ◯	T ◯ F ◯ DK ◯	T ◯ F ◯ DK ◯	**50**	T ◯ F ◯ DK ◯	T ◯ F ◯ DK ◯	T ◯ F ◯ DK ◯	T ◯ F ◯ DK ◯	T ◯ F ◯ DK ◯
36	T ◯ F ◯ DK ◯	T ◯ F ◯ DK ◯	T ◯ F ◯ DK ◯	T ◯ F ◯ DK ◯	T ◯ F ◯ DK ◯	**51**	T ◯ F ◯ DK ◯	T ◯ F ◯ DK ◯	T ◯ F ◯ DK ◯	T ◯ F ◯ DK ◯	T ◯ F ◯ DK ◯
37	T ◯ F ◯ DK ◯	T ◯ F ◯ DK ◯	T ◯ F ◯ DK ◯	T ◯ F ◯ DK ◯	T ◯ F ◯ DK ◯	**52**	T ◯ F ◯ DK ◯	T ◯ F ◯ DK ◯	T ◯ F ◯ DK ◯	T ◯ F ◯ DK ◯	T ◯ F ◯ DK ◯
38	T ◯ F ◯ DK ◯	T ◯ F ◯ DK ◯	T ◯ F ◯ DK ◯	T ◯ F ◯ DK ◯	T ◯ F ◯ DK ◯	**53**	T ◯ F ◯ DK ◯	T ◯ F ◯ DK ◯	T ◯ F ◯ DK ◯	T ◯ F ◯ DK ◯	T ◯ F ◯ DK ◯
39	T ◯ F ◯ DK ◯	T ◯ F ◯ DK ◯	T ◯ F ◯ DK ◯	T ◯ F ◯ DK ◯	T ◯ F ◯ DK ◯	**54**	T ◯ F ◯ DK ◯	T ◯ F ◯ DK ◯	T ◯ F ◯ DK ◯	T ◯ F ◯ DK ◯	T ◯ F ◯ DK ◯
40	T ◯ F ◯ DK ◯	T ◯ F ◯ DK ◯	T ◯ F ◯ DK ◯	T ◯ F ◯ DK ◯	T ◯ F ◯ DK ◯	**55**	T ◯ F ◯ DK ◯	T ◯ F ◯ DK ◯	T ◯ F ◯ DK ◯	T ◯ F ◯ DK ◯	T ◯ F ◯ DK ◯
41	T ◯ F ◯ DK ◯	T ◯ F ◯ DK ◯	T ◯ F ◯ DK ◯	T ◯ F ◯ DK ◯	T ◯ F ◯ DK ◯	**56**	T ◯ F ◯ DK ◯	T ◯ F ◯ DK ◯	T ◯ F ◯ DK ◯	T ◯ F ◯ DK ◯	T ◯ F ◯ DK ◯
42	T ◯ F ◯ DK ◯	T ◯ F ◯ DK ◯	T ◯ F ◯ DK ◯	T ◯ F ◯ DK ◯	T ◯ F ◯ DK ◯	**57**	T ◯ F ◯ DK ◯	T ◯ F ◯ DK ◯	T ◯ F ◯ DK ◯	T ◯ F ◯ DK ◯	T ◯ F ◯ DK ◯
43	T ◯ F ◯ DK ◯	T ◯ F ◯ DK ◯	T ◯ F ◯ DK ◯	T ◯ F ◯ DK ◯	T ◯ F ◯ DK ◯	**58**	T ◯ F ◯ DK ◯	T ◯ F ◯ DK ◯	T ◯ F ◯ DK ◯	T ◯ F ◯ DK ◯	T ◯ F ◯ DK ◯
44	T ◯ F ◯ DK ◯	T ◯ F ◯ DK ◯	T ◯ F ◯ DK ◯	T ◯ F ◯ DK ◯	T ◯ F ◯ DK ◯	**59**	T ◯ F ◯ DK ◯	T ◯ F ◯ DK ◯	T ◯ F ◯ DK ◯	T ◯ F ◯ DK ◯	T ◯ F ◯ DK ◯
45	T ◯ F ◯ DK ◯	T ◯ F ◯ DK ◯	T ◯ F ◯ DK ◯	T ◯ F ◯ DK ◯	T ◯ F ◯ DK ◯	**60**	T ◯ F ◯ DK ◯	T ◯ F ◯ DK ◯	T ◯ F ◯ DK ◯	T ◯ F ◯ DK ◯	T ◯ F ◯ DK ◯

1. In children, features pointing to a non-organic cause for recurrent abdominal pain are:

   a) Family history
   b) Tense personality
   c) Normal growth
   d) Pain in flanks
   e) Headaches

2. Bilateral hilar lymphadenopathy may be caused by:

   a) Hodgkin's disease
   b) Sarcoidosis
   c) Histoplasmosis
   d) Tuberculosis
   e) Berylliosis

3. Causes of migratory polyarthralgia include:

   a) Stevens Johnson syndrome
   b) Crohn's disease
   c) Whipple's disease
   d) Sarcoidosis
   e) Hepatitis B

4. Fibrous enlargement of the gums may be due to:

   a) Carbamazepine
   b) Scurvy
   c) Lead poisoning
   d) Phenytoin
   e) Sodium valproate

5. Clinical features of rheumatic fever include:

   a) Libman-Sachs endocarditis
   b) Osler's nodes
   c) Huntington's chorea
   d) Erythema marginatum
   e) Carey-Coombs murmur

6. In AIDS pneumonia:

   a) HTLV-III antibodies are often absent
   b) Mortality is 80% per episode
   c) *Pneumocystis carinii* is frequently present
   d) Cytomegalovirus is rare
   e) *Mycobacterium tuberculosis* is common

7. Which of these statement are true?

   a) Anti-idiotype antibodies occur normally
   b) IgM is a dimer
   c) Variation between antibody domains alters antigen binding
   d) C1q is a hexavalent glycoprotein
   e) IgD, like IgE, promotes mast cell degranulation

8. Which of these may cause dementia?

   a) Disseminated sclerosis
   b) Syphilis
   c) Schizophrenia
   d) Folate deficiency
   e) Pellagra

9. Features of delirium include:

   a) Auditory hallucinations
   b) Fever
   c) Word salad
   d) Depersonalisation
   e) Clouding of consciousness

10. Which of the following may cause an acute organic psychosis?

    a) Hypothyroidism
    b) Hyperthyroidism
    c) Brucellosis
    d) Scurvy
    e) Tracheomalacia

11. Which of the following are features of schizophrenia?

   a) Concrete thinking
   b) Neologisms
   c) Panic attacks
   d) Hypochondriacal delusion
   e) Visual hallucinations

12. In poliomyelitis:

   a) Muscle pain is a feature
   b) Early mobilisation is recommended
   c) Symmetrical paralysis usually occurs
   d) Paralysis continues to spread after the fever subsides
   e) Meningism is common

13. Concerning chicken pox, which are true?

   a) It is now rare because of modern vaccination
   b) Pneumonia is more common in children
   c) Rash is most marked on trunk
   d) Pox virus may be demonstrated from vesicles
   e) Encephalomyelitis may rarely occur

14. In malaria which statements are true?

   a) In quartan malaria paroxysms occur every fourth day
   b) Chloroquine prevents relapses of tertian malaria
   c) Blackwater fever occurs only with *Plasmodium malariae*
   d) *Plasmodium vivax* persists in the liver
   e) Falciparum malaria may cause cerebral and pulmonary
   disease

15. Paraquat poisoning may be associated with:

   a) Gramoxone
   b) Ulceration of the mouth
   c) Type I respiratory failure
   d) Treatment with Fuller's earth
   e) Oxygen therapy

16. Sex-linked inherited conditions include:

    a) Haemophilia A
    b) Galactosaemia
    c) Marfan's syndrome
    d) Glucose-6-phosphate dehydrogenase deficiency
    e) Kinky hair syndrome

17. Which tests are applicable to non-parametric data?

    a) Wilcoxon Rank Sum
    b) Student's paired *t*
    c) Mann-Whitney U
    d) Regression
    e) Chi-square

18. In children a ventricular septal defect:

    a) Is the commonest congenital heart lesion
    b) Closes spontaneously in up to 50% of cases
    c) Of maladie de Roger type is the most severe form
    d) Is associated with pulmonary oligaemia
    e) With a large lesion is associated with biventricular
       hypertrophy

19. Human breast milk:

    a) Can be safely used in babies with galactosaemia
    b) Contains more protein per millilitre than cow's milk
    c) Contains less fat per millilitre than cow's milk
    d) Has a relatively high sodium content
    e) Contains more carbohydrate per millilitre than cow's milk

20. Complications of kwashiorkor includes:

    a) Cardiac failure
    b) Hypoglycaemia
    c) Hypothermia
    d) Hypertrichosis
    e) Hypercalcaemia

21. By 18 months of age, a child:

    a) Can kick a ball
    b) Say up to five actual words
    c) Make a tower of six bricks
    d) Is dry by day
    e) Bangs bricks together

22. Raised unconjugated bilirubin in full-term babies:

    a) May cause opisthotonus
    b) Is dangerous below a level of 40 μmol/litre
    c) Has a greater damaging effect if albumin levels are low
    d) Is lowered by aspirin
    e) Is lipid insoluble

23. The median nerve supplies:

    a) The lateral two interossei
    b) Half flexor digitorum profundus
    c) Abductor pollicis longus
    d) Medial lumbricals
    e) Flexor pollicis brevis

24. Symptoms of hyponatraemia include:

    a) Anorexia
    b) Headache
    c) Paraesthesia
    d) Tinnitus
    e) Agitation

25. Which are true concerning body water in a 70-kg man?

    a) Total body water is 55 litres
    b) Extracellular fluid is 14 litres
    c) Plasma volume is 7 litres
    d) Intracellular fluid is 28 litres
    e) Distribution is dependent on osmolar content of various
       compartments

26. Which of the following colours of urine may be seen?

a) Orange/red — Dorbanex
b) Red — beetroot
c) Orange — isoniazid
d) Black — alkaptonuria
e) Red — myoglobinuria

27. The nephrotic syndrome may result from:

a) Bee stings
b) Renal artery stenosis
c) Chronic pyelonephritis
d) Familial hypercholesterolaemia
e) Sarcoidosis

28. Renal papillary necrosis may be due to:

a) Obstructive uropathy
b) Blackwater fever
c) Phenacitin abuse
d) Polycystic kidneys
e) Urate nephropathy

29. Pneumothorax may be caused by:

a) Acupuncture
b) Histiocytosis
c) Endometriosis
d) Rib fractures
e) Transbronchial biopsy

30. Which of the following may cause fine crepitations?

a) Sarcoidosis
b) Extrinsic allergic alveolitis
c) Bronchiectasis
d) Chronic bronchitis
e) Left ventricular failure

31. Silicosis:

    a) Is commoner in boiler scalers
    b) Causes eggshell calcification of hilar lymph nodes
    c) Rarely leads to fibrosis
    d) Causes a restrictive ventilatory defect
    e) Can cause haemoptysis

32. Hoarseness may be a feature of:

    a) Thyrotoxicosis
    b) Steroid therapy
    c) Rheumatoid arthritis
    d) Hodgkin's disease
    e) Dystrophia myotonica

33. Immediately after a large haemorrhage:

    a) Pulse pressure is increased
    b) Thirst occurs
    c) Anaerobic glycolysis increases
    d) Coronary vasoconstriction occurs
    e) Carotid chemoreceptors are inhibited

34. Hypotonia is a feature of:

    a) Syringomyelia
    b) Cerebellar degeneration
    c) Glioma of the motor cortex
    d) Poliomyelitis
    e) Dystrophia myotonica

35. Which of these can cause dementia?

    a) Motor neurone disease
    b) Nelson's syndrome
    c) Alcohol
    d) Kreutzfeld-Jacob syndrome
    e) Myxoedema

36. Which are true concerning cranial nerve supply?

   a) XI — trapezius
   b) V — muscles of mastication
   c) VII — taste, posterior third of tongue
   d) III — levator palpebrae superioris
   e) IV — lateral rectus

37. Ptosis may result from:

   a) Disseminated sclerosis
   b) Parasympathetic lesions
   c) Syringomyelia
   d) Diabetes mellitus
   e) Myasthenia gravis

38. Horner's syndrome may be caused by:

   a) Posterior communicating artery aneurysm
   b) Posterior inferior cerebellar artery occlusion
   c) Syphilis
   d) C6 osteolytic lesion
   e) Carotid artery aneurysm

39. Complications of Behçet's syndrome include:

   a) Thrombophlebitis
   b) Ulcerative colitis
   c) Erythema marginatum
   d) Retrobulbar neuritis
   e) Hyperuricaemia

40. In psoriatic arthropathy:

   a) HLA-B27 is positive
   b) Severity of the arthropathy is related to severity of the
      psoriaris
   c) Use of PUVA is contraindicated for skin lesions
   d) Nail pitting is always present
   e) Arthritis mutilans is a feature

41. Which of the following may affect T cell immunity?

    a) Angio-oedema
    b) Wiskott-Aldrich syndrome
    c) Measles
    d) DiGeorge syndrome
    e) Ataxia telangiectasia

42. Iron deficiency anaemia:

    a) Is rare in the Mallory-Weiss syndrome
    b) Is commonly caused by rheumatoid arthritis
    c) Is common in haemophilia
    d) Initially responds to folate replacement
    e) Causes target cells in the peripheral blood

43. Which of the following are causes of macrocytic anaemia?

    a) Rheumatoid arthritis
    b) Isoniazid therapy
    c) Thalassaemia minor
    d) Myelomatosis
    e) Lead poisoning

44. Polycythaemia may be caused by:

    a) A raised carboxyhaemoglobin
    b) Hyperparathyroidism
    c) Phaeochromocytoma
    d) Haemochromatosis
    e) Hepatoma

45. Which of the following are recognised associations with coeliac disease?

    a) Temporal lobe epilepsy
    b) Milk intolerance
    c) Hashimoto's thyroiditis
    d) Hyposplenism
    e) Gastric lymphoma

46. Achlorhydria may result from:

    a) Wilson's disease
    b) Pernicious anaemia
    c) Giardiasis
    d) Pellagra
    e) Ulcerative colitis

47. In the oesophagus:

    a) Striated muscle ends at the junction of upper and middle thirds
    b) The lower end is anchored by the phreno-oesophageal ligament
    c) Stratified squamous epithelium is usually found until the level of the diaphragm
    d) Pressure in the lower oesophagus may reach 500 mmHg
    e) Alcohol increases lower oesophageal tone

48. Which of the following may be radio-opaque on a plain abdominal X-ray?

    a) Hepatoma
    b) Slow-K tablets
    c) Urate stone
    d) Faecolith
    e) Histoplasmosis of the liver

49. Which of the following are signs of digoxin toxicity?

    a) Supraventricular tachycardia
    b) Bradycardia
    c) Short QT interval
    d) Loss of appetite
    e) Teichopsia

50. Which of the following drugs are recognised causes of pulmonary fibrosis?

    a) Penicillamine
    b) Busulphan
    c) Methotrexate
    d) Prednisolone
    e) Sulphamethoxazole

51. Which of the following are side-effects of gold therapy?

a) Neutropenia
b) Heavy chain disease
c) Proteinuria
d) Fixed drug eruption
e) Jaundice

52. Which of the following are hepatic enzyme inducers?

a) Trimethoprim
b) Phenytoin
c) Temazepam
d) Rifampicin
e) Ampicillin

53. Drugs which reduce renal concentrating ability include:

a) Amoxycillin
b) Lithium
c) Tetracycline
d) Salbutamol
e) Amphotericin B

54. Gynaecomastia may occur in:

a) Patients with pituitary failure
b) Chronic renal failure
c) Paraplegia
d) Amiodarone treatment
e) Isoniazid treatment

55. In ovulation:

a) The granulosa cells proliferate in response to raised progestogens
b) Many graafian follicles mature
c) An increase in oestradiol leads to a rise in luteinising hormone secretion
d) The corpus luteum usually atrophies after 10 days if fertilisation fails
e) Follicular stimulating hormone peaks twice

56. Senile osteoporosis is associated with:

a) Myeloma
b) Calcitonin therapy
c) Improvement with 1,25-dihydroxy cholecalciferol therapy
d) A delayed menopause
e) Haemochromatosis

57. Nail pitting may occur in:

a) Lichen planus
b) Dermatomyositis
c) Alopecia
d) Pachydermoperiostitis
e) Acromegaly

58. Which may cause pulmonary hypertension?

a) Coarctation of the aorta
b) Pulmonary stenosis
c) Patent ductus arteriosus
d) Kyphoscoliosis
e) Schistosomiasis

59. Major determinants of myocardial oxygen requirements include:

a) Left ventricular diastolic pressure
b) Heart size
c) Coronary artery patency
d) Heart rate
e) Left atrial pressure

60. Reverse splitting of the 2nd heart sound

a) Occurs in right bundle branch block
b) Occurs in aortic stenosis
c) Occurs in systolic hypertension
d) Occurs in mitral regurgitation
e) Is more easily heard on inspiration

Examination 3

All parts of every Question
must be answered *True* or *False*
or *Don't Know* by filling in the
box provided. Failure to do so
will result in rejection of the
answer sheet

SURNAME

INITIALS

Please use 2B PENCIL only. Rub out all errors thoroughly.
Mark lozenges like ● NOT like this ⌀ ⌀ ⌀

T ⊂⊃ = TRUE   F ⊂⊃ = FALSE   DK ⊂⊃ = DON'T KNOW

	A	B	C	D	E		A	B	C	D	E
1	T F DK	T F DK	T F DK	T F DK	T F DK	16	T F DK	T F DK	T F DK	T F DK	T F DK
2	T F DK	T F DK	T F DK	T F DK	T F DK	17	T F DK	T F DK	T F DK	T F DK	T F DK
3	T F DK	T F DK	T F DK	T F DK	T F DK	18	T F DK	T F DK	T F DK	T F DK	T F DK
4	T F DK	T F DK	T F DK	T F DK	T F DK	19	T F DK	T F DK	T F DK	T F DK	T F DK
5	T F DK	T F DK	T F DK	T F DK	T F DK	20	T F DK	T F DK	T F DK	T F DK	T F DK
6	T F DK	T F DK	T F DK	T F DK	T F DK	21	T F DK	T F DK	T F DK	T F DK	T F DK
7	T F DK	T F DK	T F DK	T F DK	T F DK	22	T F DK	T F DK	T F DK	T F DK	T F DK
8	T F DK	T F DK	T F DK	T F DK	T F DK	23	T F DK	T F DK	T F DK	T F DK	T F DK
9	T F DK	T F DK	T F DK	T F DK	T F DK	24	T F DK	T F DK	T F DK	T F DK	T F DK
10	T F DK	T F DK	T F DK	T F DK	T F DK	25	T F DK	T F DK	T F DK	T F DK	T F DK
11	T F DK	T F DK	T F DK	T F DK	T F DK	26	T F DK	T F DK	T F DK	T F DK	T F DK
12	T F DK	T F DK	T F DK	T F DK	T F DK	27	T F DK	T F DK	T F DK	T F DK	T F DK
13	T F DK	T F DK	T F DK	T F DK	T F DK	28	T F DK	T F DK	T F DK	T F DK	T F DK
14	T F DK	T F DK	T F DK	T F DK	T F DK	29	T F DK	T F DK	T F DK	T F DK	T F DK
15	T F DK	T F DK	T F DK	T F DK	T F DK	30	T F DK	T F DK	T F DK	T F DK	T F DK

	A	B	C	D	E			A	B	C	D	E
31	T F DK	T F DK	T F DK	T F DK	T F DK		**46**	T F DK	T F DK	T F DK	T F DK	T F DK
32	T F DK	T F DK	T F DK	T F DK	T F DK		**47**	T F DK	T F DK	T F DK	T F DK	T F DK
33	T F DK	T F DK	T F DK	T F DK	T F DK		**48**	T F DK	T F DK	T F DK	T F DK	T F DK
34	T F DK	T F DK	T F DK	T F DK	T F DK		**49**	T F DK	T F DK	T F DK	T F DK	T F DK
35	T F DK	T F DK	T F DK	T F DK	T F DK		**50**	T F DK	T F DK	T F DK	T F DK	T F DK
36	T F DK	T F DK	T F DK	T F DK	T F DK		**51**	T F DK	T F DK	T F DK	T F DK	T F DK
37	T F DK	T F DK	T F DK	T F DK	T F DK		**52**	T F DK	T F DK	T F DK	T F DK	T F DK
38	T F DK	T F DK	T F DK	T F DK	T F DK		**53**	T F DK	T F DK	T F DK	T F DK	T F DK
39	T F DK	T F DK	T F DK	T F DK	T F DK		**54**	T F DK	T F DK	T F DK	T F DK	T F DK
40	T F DK	T F DK	T F DK	T F DK	T F DK		**55**	T F DK	T F DK	T F DK	T F DK	T F DK
41	T F DK	T F DK	T F DK	T F DK	T F DK		**56**	T F DK	T F DK	T F DK	T F DK	T F DK
42	T F DK	T F DK	T F DK	T F DK	T F DK		**57**	T F DK	T F DK	T F DK	T F DK	T F DK
43	T F DK	T F DK	T F DK	T F DK	T F DK		**58**	T F DK	T F DK	T F DK	T F DK	T F DK
44	T F DK	T F DK	T F DK	T F DK	T F DK		**59**	T F DK	T F DK	T F DK	T F DK	T F DK
45	T F DK	T F DK	T F DK	T F DK	T F DK		**60**	T F DK	T F DK	T F DK	T F DK	T F DK

1. Chloroquine may be used in:

   a) Senile macular degeneration
   b) Amoebic liver abscess
   c) Lichen planus
   d) Discoid lupus
   e) Rheumatoid arthritis

2. Which of the following drugs undergo enterohepatic circulation?

   a) Rifampicin
   b) Digoxin
   c) Oestrogen
   d) Thyroxine
   e) Phenytoin

3. Which of the following drugs are excreted in breast milk and produce adverse effects on nursing infants?

   a) Ergot alkaloids
   b) Diazepam
   c) Morphine
   d) Atropine
   e) Iodides

4. Causes of excessively tall children include:

   a) Thyrotoxicosis
   b) Soto's syndrome
   c) Pyruvate kinase deficiency
   d) Homocystinuria
   e) Arrhenoblastoma

5. Which statements concerning the anatomy of the lung are true?

   a) The right upper lobe divides into three segments
   b) The left main bronchus is straighter than the right
   c) The trachea bifurcates at the angle of Louis
   d) The bronchial arteries arise from the aorta
   e) The lingula has three segmental bronchi

6. Eye disease in sarcoidosis includes:

   a) Retinal neovascularisation
   b) Posterior uveitis
   c) Anterior uveitis
   d) Band keratopathy
   e) Pigmented maculopathy

7. Rubella embryopathy is characterised by:

   a) A maculopapular rash
   b) Deafness
   c) Spinal cord anomalies
   d) Cataracts
   e) Excretion of live virus for several months after birth

8. In head injury, the period of post-traumatic amnesia is correlated with:

   a) The severity of any memory deficit
   b) The severity of generalised intellectual impairment
   c) The severity of any personality change
   d) The severity of physical injury
   e) The period of retrograde amnesia

9. Psychiatric effects of frontal lobe lesions include:

   a) Disinhibition
   b) Over-talkativeness
   c) Depression
   d) Visuo-spatial difficulties
   e) Severe intellectual deficit

10. Paranoid schizophrenia:

    a) Occurs in the younger age group
    b) Delusions occur which change from day to day
    c) Auditory hallucinations unrelated to the delusions are a feature
    d) Visual hallucinations are a feature
    e) Guilt and retardation are marked

11. Schneider's front rank symptoms of schizophrenia include:

    a) Thought broadcasting
    b) Delusional perception
    c) Bodily hallucination
    d) Euphoria
    e) Guilt

12. The following infections may cause hepatitis:

    a) Lassa fever
    b) Argentinian haemorrhagic fever
    c) Herpes hominis
    d) Ebola virus
    e) Influenza A

13. In idiopathic haemachromatosis:

    a) The total body iron is high
    b) Iron absorption from the gastrointestinal tract is relatively
       normal
    c) HLA B14 is found with a high frequency
    d) Iron excess can be found in the synovia
    e) Pigmentation is due to excess iron in the skin

14. Normal bile:

    a) Is hypertonic
    b) Has a high protein content
    c) Contains phospholipid
    d) Contains unesterified cholesterol
    e) Output is 125 ml/24 hours

15. Which of the following renal stones are radiolucent?

    a) Magnesium ammonium phosphate
    b) Matrix
    c) Calcium oxalate
    d) Xanthine
    e) Calcium phosphate

16. Potentially reversible causes of chronic renal failure include:

    a) Chronic glomerulonephritis
    b) Subacute bacterial endocarditis
    c) Polycystic kidneys
    d) Urinary tract obstruction
    e) Hyperuricaemia

17. Indications for dialysis in renal failure include:

    a) Poorly controlled diabetes mellitus
    b) Arterial pH of greater than 7.25
    c) Water overload
    d) Serum potassium of 7.5 mmol/litre
    e) Rapidly rising blood urea

18. Inability of tubular resorption of glucose occurs in:

    a) Hypercalcaemia
    b) Primary renal tubular acidosis
    c) Myelomatosis
    d) Heavy metal poisoning
    e) Hartnup disease

19. Causes of a serum paraprotein include:

    a) Chronic lymphocytic leukaemia
    b) Chronic cold haemagglutinin disease
    c) Acute myeloid leukaemia
    d) Malignant lymphoma
    e) Chronic folate deficiency

20. Which of the following are features of diabetic autonomic neuropathy?

    a) Impotence
    b) Cardiorespiratory arrest
    c) Dependent oedema
    d) Hyperhidrosis
    e) Constipation

21. Which are true?

   a) The standard deviation is the square root of the variance
   b) Only 5% of values fall above the 95% confidence limit
   c) Yates correction should be applied to Wilcoxon's test if
      there are small numbers
   d) Using Student's *t*-test with ten paired observations there are
      19 degrees of freedom
   e) Chi-squared tests can only be carried out on means of
      observations

22. Cow's milk protein intolerance may cause:

   a) Stridor
   b) Bloody diarrhoea
   c) Flat jejunal villi
   d) Soya protein intolerance
   e) Acrodermatitis enteropathica

23. In childhood measles:

   a) The incubation period is 7 days
   b) Conjunctivitis occurs late in the disease
   c) The rash appears on the 2nd day
   d) Otitis media is common
   e) Koplik's spots are unusual

24. Which of the following are causes of nephrocalcinosis?

   a) Milk alkali syndrome
   b) Sarcoidosis
   c) Renal tubular acidosis
   d) Histoplasmosis
   e) Hyperparathyroidism

25. Which of the following may cause a phrenic nerve palsy?

   a) Aortic aneurysm
   b) Pericardial cyst
   c) Dermoid
   d) Ganglioneuroma
   e) Sarcoidosis

26. Cystic fibrosis is associated with:

    a) Decreased sweat sodium
    b) Pseudomonal infection
    c) Autosomal dominant inheritance
    d) Rectal prolapse
    e) Retroperitoneal fibrosis

27. A $PaCO_2$ of 60 mmHg (8 kPa) may be caused by:

    a) Chronic renal failure
    b) Chronic bronchitis
    c) Early cryptogenic fibrosing alveolitis
    d) Acute pneumonia
    e) Mild asthma

28. Which of the following provide part of the control mechanism for respiration in man?

    a) Venous HCO_3
    b) CSF pH
    c) CSF $PaCO_2$
    d) Arterial PO_2
    e) Arterial PCO_2

29. Mononeuritis multiplex results from:

    a) Rothman's syndrome
    b) Gaucher's disease
    c) Polyarteritis nodosum
    d) Tay Sachs disease
    e) Leprosy

30. Which of the following may present with epilepsy?

    a) Subdural haematoma
    b) Alkalosis
    c) Paragonimiasis
    d) Hypertension
    e) Cadmium poisoning

31. Myasthenia gravis may be associated with:

a) A remission in pregnancy
b) Hyperthyroidism
c) Oat cell carcinoma of the bronchus
d) A low FEV_1
e) Small cell tumour of the thymus

32. Carotenaemia occurs in:

a) An excess of mangoes in the diet
b) Addison's disease
c) Hyperbetalipoproteinaemia
d) Biliary atresia
e) Myxoedema

33. Hypokalaemia may occur in:

a) Bartter's syndrome
b) Liver failure
c) Conn's syndrome
d) Treatment with amphotericin B
e) Thyrotoxic periodic paralysis

34. Which of the following may occur in the respiratory tract in rheumatoid arthritis?

a) Tracheomalacia
b) Bronchiolitis
c) Cavitating mass lesions
d) Bronchial hyper-reactivity
e) Hilar lymphadenopathy

35. Associations of gout include:

a) Calcaneal spur
b) Sacroiliitis
c) Renal colic
d) Olecranon bursitis
e) Sjögren's syndrome

36. Which of the following are clinical features of Behçet's syndrome

a) Oral bullae
b) Thrombophlebitis
c) Keratoderma blennorrhagicum
d) Circinate balanitis
e) Hypopyon

37. Dactylitis may occur in:

a) Sickle cell anaemia
b) Sarcoidosis
c) Tuberculosis
d) Psoriasis
e) Gout

38. Which of the following may impair T-lymphocyte responses?

a) Plasma exchange
b) Antilymphocyte serum
c) Alpha interferon
d) Niridazole
e) Aspirin

39. Hypersplenism may result from:

a) Sarcoidosis
b) Brucellosis
c) Beta-thalassaemia major
d) Coeliac disease
e) Hodgkin's disease

40. In which of the following anaemias is the reticulocyte count elevated?

a) The anaemia of chronic infection
b) Paroxysmal nocturnal haemoglobinuria
c) Sideroblastic anaemia
d) G6PD deficiency
e) Sickle cell disease

41. Which of the following may present with angular stomatitis?

   a) Aphthous ulcer
   b) Syphilis
   c) Iron deficiency
   d) Psoriasis
   e) Reiter's disease

42. Which of the following may cause a bullous rash?

   a) Arsenic
   b) Sulphonamides
   c) Bromides
   d) Barbiturates
   e) Hydralazine

43. Which of these drugs should be avoided in breast-feeding mothers?

   a) Carbimazole
   b) Benzodiazepines
   c) Chloramphenicol
   d) Gentamicin
   e) Labetalol

44. A fat embolism:

   a) Is usually fatal
   b) May be associated with a skin rash
   c) Causes fat in the urine
   d) Causes a rise in $PaCO_2$
   e) Causes a fall in PaO_2

45. In juvenile onset diabetes mellitus:

   a) Pancreatic islet cell antibodies are common
   b) Diet is the therapy of choice
   c) Arterial complications are rare
   d) Beta-blockers are useful in treating hypoglycaemic symptoms
   e) Insulin antibodies are the cause of the disease

46. Hypoglycaemia may result from:

    a) Diazoxide therapy
    b) Alcohol abuse
    c) Marathon running
    d) Addison's disease
    e) Carcinoma of the pancreas

47. Increased concentrations of thyroid binding globulin (TBG) are found in:

    a) Chronic liver disease
    b) Acromegaly
    c) Pregnancy
    d) Oral contraceptive therapy
    e) Acute hepatitis

48. Which of the following conditions are associated with malignancy?

    a) Geographical tongue
    b) Acanthosis nigricans
    c) Lichen planus
    d) Hypertrichosis lanugosa
    e) Erythema gyratum repens

49. Which of the following conditions may lead to high output cardiac failure?

    a) Aortic stenosis
    b) Beri-Beri
    c) Gram-negative sepsis
    d) Paget's disease
    e) Two vessel coronary artery disease

50. Low T-waves on an ECG result from:

    a) Hypokalaemia
    b) Addison's disease
    c) Pericardial effusion
    d) Thyrotoxicosis
    e) Pernicious anaemia

51. Which of the following are determinants of preload?

    a) Venous tone
    b) Capillary tone
    c) Total blood volume
    d) Blood pressure
    e) Atrial contraction

52. A continuous murmur in systole and diastole may be heard with:

    a) Atrial septal defect and ventricular septal defect
    b) Aortic stenosis and aortic incompetence
    c) Patent ductus arteriosus
    d) Mitral stenosis and aortic incompetence
    e) Pulmonary AV fistula

53. Which of these statements concerning the second heart sound is true?

    a) Paradoxical split in right bundle branch block
    b) Loud with narrow split in an atrial septal defect
    c) Normally splits on inspiration
    d) Soft and widely split in pulmonary stenosis
    e) P_2 precedes A_2 in the Eisenmenger syndrome

54. For which of these diseases is a live attenuated vaccine available?

    a) Smallpox
    b) Poliomyelitis
    c) AIDS
    d) Hepatitis B
    e) Typhoid

55. The WR may be positive in:

    a) Yaws
    b) Cat scratch fever
    c) Systemic lupus erythematosus
    d) Hashimoto's thyroiditis
    e) Sarcoidosis

56. Which of the following infective organisms are common pathogens in patients with the acquired immune deficiency syndrome?

   a) *Toxoplasma gondii*
   b) Coxsackie A virus
   c) Herpes simplex
   d) *Pneumocystis carinii*
   e) Pneumococcus

57. Which of these are DNA viruses?

   a) Herpes simplex
   b) Polio
   c) Influenza A
   d) Vaccinia
   e) EB virus

58. A metabolic acidosis may result from:

   a) Hepatic coma
   b) Type II respiratory failure
   c) Gram-negative sepsis
   d) Laxative abuse
   e) Myocardial infarction

59. Erythema nodosum may be caused by:

   a) SLE
   b) Contraceptive pill
   c) Trimethoprim
   d) Sarcoidosis
   e) Besnier's prurigo

60. Hyperuricaemia may result from:

   a) Hypoadrenalism
   b) Psoriasis
   c) Hyperparathyroidism
   d) Chronic renal failure
   e) Porphyria cutanea tarda

Examination 4

All parts of every Question must be answered *True* or *False* or *Don't Know* by filling in the box provided. Failure to do so will result in rejection of the answer sheet

✂

EXAMINATION NO.

4

SURNAME

INITIALS

Please use 2B PENCIL only. Rub out all errors thoroughly.
Mark lozenges like ▬ <u>NOT</u> like this ⌀ ⌀ ⌀

T ◯ = TRUE   F ◯ = FALSE   DK ◯ = DON'T KNOW

	A	B	C	D	E		A	B	C	D	E
1	T F DK	T F DK	T F DK	T F DK	T F DK	16	T F DK	T F DK	T F DK	T F DK	T F DK
2	T F DK	T F DK	T F DK	T F DK	T F DK	17	T F DK	T F DK	T F DK	T F DK	T F DK
3	T F DK	T F DK	T F DK	T F DK	T F DK	18	T F DK	T F DK	T F DK	T F DK	T F DK
4	T F DK	T F DK	T F DK	T F DK	T F DK	19	T F DK	T F DK	T F DK	T F DK	T F DK
5	T F DK	T F DK	T F DK	T F DK	T F DK	20	T F DK	T F DK	T F DK	T F DK	T F DK
6	T F DK	T F DK	T F DK	T F DK	T F DK	21	T F DK	T F DK	T F DK	T F DK	T F DK
7	T F DK	T F DK	T F DK	T F DK	T F DK	22	T F DK	T F DK	T F DK	T F DK	T F DK
8	T F DK	T F DK	T F DK	T F DK	T F DK	23	T F DK	T F DK	T F DK	T F DK	T F DK
9	T F DK	T F DK	T F DK	T F DK	T F DK	24	T F DK	T F DK	T F DK	T F DK	T F DK
10	T F DK	T F DK	T F DK	T F DK	T F DK	25	T F DK	T F DK	T F DK	T F DK	T F DK
11	T F DK	T F DK	T F DK	T F DK	T F DK	26	T F DK	T F DK	T F DK	T F DK	T F DK
12	T F DK	T F DK	T F DK	T F DK	T F DK	27	T F DK	T F DK	T F DK	T F DK	T F DK
13	T F DK	T F DK	T F DK	T F DK	T F DK	28	T F DK	T F DK	T F DK	T F DK	T F DK
14	T F DK	T F DK	T F DK	T F DK	T F DK	29	T F DK	T F DK	T F DK	T F DK	T F DK
15	T F DK	T F DK	T F DK	T F DK	T F DK	30	T F DK	T F DK	T F DK	T F DK	T F DK

	A	B	C	D	E		A	B	C	D	E
31	T ☐ F ☐ DK ☐	T ☐ F ☐ DK ☐	T ☐ F ☐ DK ☐	T ☐ F ☐ DK ☐	T ☐ F ☐ DK ☐	46	T ☐ F ☐ DK ☐	T ☐ F ☐ DK ☐	T ☐ F ☐ DK ☐	T ☐ F ☐ DK ☐	T ☐ F ☐ DK ☐
32	T ☐ F ☐ DK ☐	T ☐ F ☐ DK ☐	T ☐ F ☐ DK ☐	T ☐ F ☐ DK ☐	T ☐ F ☐ DK ☐	47	T ☐ F ☐ DK ☐	T ☐ F ☐ DK ☐	T ☐ F ☐ DK ☐	T ☐ F ☐ DK ☐	T ☐ F ☐ DK ☐
33	T ☐ F ☐ DK ☐	T ☐ F ☐ DK ☐	T ☐ F ☐ DK ☐	T ☐ F ☐ DK ☐	T ☐ F ☐ DK ☐	48	T ☐ F ☐ DK ☐	T ☐ F ☐ DK ☐	T ☐ F ☐ DK ☐	T ☐ F ☐ DK ☐	T ☐ F ☐ DK ☐
34	T ☐ F ☐ DK ☐	T ☐ F ☐ DK ☐	T ☐ F ☐ DK ☐	T ☐ F ☐ DK ☐	T ☐ F ☐ DK ☐	49	T ☐ F ☐ DK ☐	T ☐ F ☐ DK ☐	T ☐ F ☐ DK ☐	T ☐ F ☐ DK ☐	T ☐ F ☐ DK ☐
35	T ☐ F ☐ DK ☐	T ☐ F ☐ DK ☐	T ☐ F ☐ DK ☐	T ☐ F ☐ DK ☐	T ☐ F ☐ DK ☐	50	T ☐ F ☐ DK ☐	T ☐ F ☐ DK ☐	T ☐ F ☐ DK ☐	T ☐ F ☐ DK ☐	T ☐ F ☐ DK ☐
36	T ☐ F ☐ DK ☐	T ☐ F ☐ DK ☐	T ☐ F ☐ DK ☐	T ☐ F ☐ DK ☐	T ☐ F ☐ DK ☐	51	T ☐ F ☐ DK ☐	T ☐ F ☐ DK ☐	T ☐ F ☐ DK ☐	T ☐ F ☐ DK ☐	T ☐ F ☐ DK ☐
37	T ☐ F ☐ DK ☐	T ☐ F ☐ DK ☐	T ☐ F ☐ DK ☐	T ☐ F ☐ DK ☐	T ☐ F ☐ DK ☐	52	T ☐ F ☐ DK ☐	T ☐ F ☐ DK ☐	T ☐ F ☐ DK ☐	T ☐ F ☐ DK ☐	T ☐ F ☐ DK ☐
38	T ☐ F ☐ DK ☐	T ☐ F ☐ DK ☐	T ☐ F ☐ DK ☐	T ☐ F ☐ DK ☐	T ☐ F ☐ DK ☐	53	T ☐ F ☐ DK ☐	T ☐ F ☐ DK ☐	T ☐ F ☐ DK ☐	T ☐ F ☐ DK ☐	T ☐ F ☐ DK ☐
39	T ☐ F ☐ DK ☐	T ☐ F ☐ DK ☐	T ☐ F ☐ DK ☐	T ☐ F ☐ DK ☐	T ☐ F ☐ DK ☐	54	T ☐ F ☐ DK ☐	T ☐ F ☐ DK ☐	T ☐ F ☐ DK ☐	T ☐ F ☐ DK ☐	T ☐ F ☐ DK ☐
40	T ☐ F ☐ DK ☐	T ☐ F ☐ DK ☐	T ☐ F ☐ DK ☐	T ☐ F ☐ DK ☐	T ☐ F ☐ DK ☐	55	T ☐ F ☐ DK ☐	T ☐ F ☐ DK ☐	T ☐ F ☐ DK ☐	T ☐ F ☐ DK ☐	T ☐ F ☐ DK ☐
41	T ☐ F ☐ DK ☐	T ☐ F ☐ DK ☐	T ☐ F ☐ DK ☐	T ☐ F ☐ DK ☐	T ☐ F ☐ DK ☐	56	T ☐ F ☐ DK ☐	T ☐ F ☐ DK ☐	T ☐ F ☐ DK ☐	T ☐ F ☐ DK ☐	T ☐ F ☐ DK ☐
42	T ☐ F ☐ DK ☐	T ☐ F ☐ DK ☐	T ☐ F ☐ DK ☐	T ☐ F ☐ DK ☐	T ☐ F ☐ DK ☐	57	T ☐ F ☐ DK ☐	T ☐ F ☐ DK ☐	T ☐ F ☐ DK ☐	T ☐ F ☐ DK ☐	T ☐ F ☐ DK ☐
43	T ☐ F ☐ DK ☐	T ☐ F ☐ DK ☐	T ☐ F ☐ DK ☐	T ☐ F ☐ DK ☐	T ☐ F ☐ DK ☐	58	T ☐ F ☐ DK ☐	T ☐ F ☐ DK ☐	T ☐ F ☐ DK ☐	T ☐ F ☐ DK ☐	T ☐ F ☐ DK ☐
44	T ☐ F ☐ DK ☐	T ☐ F ☐ DK ☐	T ☐ F ☐ DK ☐	T ☐ F ☐ DK ☐	T ☐ F ☐ DK ☐	59	T ☐ F ☐ DK ☐	T ☐ F ☐ DK ☐	T ☐ F ☐ DK ☐	T ☐ F ☐ DK ☐	T ☐ F ☐ DK ☐
45	T ☐ F ☐ DK ☐	T ☐ F ☐ DK ☐	T ☐ F ☐ DK ☐	T ☐ F ☐ DK ☐	T ☐ F ☐ DK ☐	60	T ☐ F ☐ DK ☐	T ☐ F ☐ DK ☐	T ☐ F ☐ DK ☐	T ☐ F ☐ DK ☐	T ☐ F ☐ DK ☐

1. Bromocriptine:

   a) Will suppress lactation in the puerperium
   b) May be a useful adjunct in acromegaly
   c) May cause enlargement of the pituitary in a patient with a prolactinoma
   d) Inhibits dopamine receptors
   e) Is an ergot derivative

2. The following are normal findings in children:

   a) Standing unaided at 13 months
   b) First lower molars erupting at age 6 months
   c) Extensor plantar response at age 26 months
   d) Can say four words at age 24 months
   e) Control of bowels by age 13 months

3. Phenylketonuria is associated with:

   a) Eczematous skin lesions
   b) Mental subnormality
   c) Shagreen patches
   d) Strawberry naevi
   e) Phenylalanine hydroxylase deficiency

4. Bereavement reactions may include:

   a) Lack of emotional reaction
   b) Motor restlessness
   c) Hallucinations
   d) Word salad
   e) Thought withdrawal

5. With solvent abuse:

   a) Ataxia occurs
   b) Hallucinations, usually visual in nature, occur
   c) Intoxication is short lived
   d) A peripheral neuropathy may result
   e) Females are more frequent abusers than males

6. The following parasites commonly cause diarrhoea in infected hosts:

   a) *Isospora hominis*
   b) *Cryptosporidia*
   c) *Ascaris lumbricoides*
   d) *Giardia lamblia*
   e) *Capillaria philippinensis*

7. In senile dementia of the Alzheimer type:

   a) Increased fibrous gliosis and neuro-fibrillary tangles are seen in the brain
   b) Multiple infarcts are characteristic
   c) Reduced levels of acetylcholinesterase have been reported
   d) Localised cerebral atrophy occurs
   e) Loss of sphincter control is an early feature of the disease

8. Which of these statements concerning non-A non-B hepatitis are true?

   a) The commonest cause is blood transfusion
   b) It causes about 2% of sporadic acute hepatitis in the Western world
   c) The incubation period is greater than 3 weeks
   d) A chronic carrier state does not occur
   e) Immune serum globulin is of no protective benefit to contacts

9. The following complications of ulcerative colitis often improve after colectomy:

   a) Fistulae
   b) Pyoderma gangrenosum
   c) Iritis
   d) Arthritis
   e) Cirrhosis

10. Which of the following are recognised causes of a large kidney?

   a) Chronic pyelonephritis
   b) Hydronephrosis
   c) Nephrotic syndrome
   d) Contralateral nephrectomy
   e) Bilateral renal artery stenosis

11. Which of the following conditions may cause jaundice and renal failure?

   a) Paracetamol poisoning
   b) Aspirin poisoning
   c) Mismatched blood transfusions
   d) Weil's disease
   e) Primary biliary cirrhosis

12. Continuous ambulatory peritoneal dialysis:

   a) Requires strict dietary restriction
   b) Is associated with a high incidence of renal osteo-dystrophy
   c) Requires extensive modification of the patient's home
   d) Is unsuitable for the elderly
   e) Involves only a low risk of peritonitis

13. Selective neutropenia may be due to which of the following causes?

   a) Treatment with chlorpromazine
   b) Treatment with carbimazole
   c) A familial trait
   d) Miliary tuberculosis
   e) Treatment with phenytoin

14. Which of the following are contraindications for electroconvulsive therapy?

   a) Epilepsy
   b) Atrial fibrillation
   c) A patient over 65 years
   d) Osteoporosis of the lumbar spine
   e) Dementia

15. In antithrombin III deficiency:

   a) The inheritance is autosomal recessive
   b) Thromboembolism commencing in pregnancy is common
   c) Long-term heparinisation is the treatment of choice
   d) Antithrombin III levels of 45% may predispose to embolus
   e) The presence of lupus anticoagulant is a common associated feature

16. Common features of normal pressure hydrocephalus are:

    a) Papilloedema
    b) Headache
    c) Ataxia
    d) Incontinence
    e) Disorientation

17. Which are true?

    a) Wilcoxon's rank test needs equal sample sizes
    b) Correlation coefficients vary between $+10$ and -10
    c) Student's t-test is a non-parametric test
    d) t is the symbol denoting coefficient of correlation
    e) $y = a + bx$ is a regression equation

18. Which of the following are autosomal recessive disorders?

    a) Myotonic dystrophy
    b) Wilson's disease
    c) Colour blindness
    d) Cystic fibrosis
    e) Beta-thalassaemia

19. Which of the following are characteristic of advanced fibrosing alveolitis?

    a) Increased static compliance
    b) Pleuritic chest pain
    c) Increased residual volume
    d) Cyanosis on exertion
    e) Ventilation perfusion mismatch

20. The gas transfer (DLCO) depends on:

    a) The volume of the pulmonary capillary bed
    b) Ventilation/perfusion matching
    c) The calibre of small airways
    d) Haemoglobin concentration
    e) Residual volume

21. In oat cell carcinoma of the bronchus which of these statements is true?

a) Surgery is rarely possible
b) There is no relationship to smoking
c) Chemotherapy prolongs median survival to 2 years
d) Cerebral secondaries occur more rarely than with other cell types of lung cancer
e) The tumour is usually resistant to radiotherapy

22. Cyanosis may be apparent with:

a) Oxygen saturations of less than 85%
b) Beta-thalassaemia major
c) Sickle cell crisis
d) Methaemoglobinaemia
e) Carbon monoxide poisoning

23. Which of the following may cause epilepsy?

a) Hypernatraemia
b) Hypothermia
c) Sturge-Weber syndrome
d) Doxapram infusion
e) Hyponatraemia

24. The following are features of the Ramsay-Hunt syndrome:

a) Corneal ulceration
b) Pain in the ear
c) Loss of taste over the posterior third of tongue
d) Unilateral facial paralysis, including the forehead
e) Unilateral facial hemianaesthesia

25. Optic atrophy may result from:

a) Methyl alcohol
b) Paget's disease
c) Ethambutol
d) Papilloedema
e) Tobacco

26. Signs of posterior inferior cerebellar artery thrombosis include:

    a) Ipsilateral 5th nerve sensory loss
    b) Nystagmus to the side of the lesion
    c) Contralateral loss of pain in limbs and trunk
    d) Bulbar palsy
    e) Transient ipsilateral 6th, 7th or 8th nerve palsy

27. Features of water intoxication are:

    a) Peripheral oedema
    b) Restlessness
    c) Muscular cramps
    d) Flapping tremor
    e) Cerebral oedema

28. In patients with water deprivation:

    a) Food intake is increased
    b) ADH secretion is increased
    c) Thirst-sensitive areas in the limbic centre are triggered
    d) Urine specific gravity rises
    e) A 1% change in body osmolality can be detected by the hypothalamus

29. In ochronosis:

    a) Homogentisic acid crystals are deposited in joints
    b) Calcification of cartilage occurs
    c) Acidification of urine turns it black
    d) The hands are spared
    e) The sclera are affected

30. Hypermobility is associated with:

    a) Hyperlysinaemia
    b) Tabes dorsalis
    c) Homocystinuria
    d) Rheumatoid arthritis
    e) Osteogenesis imperfecta

31. In ankylosing spondylitis:

 a) Upper lobe fibrosis of the lung may occur
 b) Most are HLA DW2 positive
 c) Radiotherapy may be useful
 d) Aortitis may occur
 e) Anterior lens dislocation occurs

32. Which of the following are well recognised side-effects of gold therapy for rheumatoid arthritis?

 a) Fixed drug eruptions
 b) Eighth nerve damage
 c) Proteinuria
 d) Hepatitis
 e) Retroperitoneal fibrosis

33. Fc receptors are found on:

 a) Neutrophils
 b) Monocytes
 c) Alveolar macrophages
 d) B-lymphocytes
 e) Platelets

34. Target cells may result from:

 a) Splenectomy
 b) Sickle cell anaemia
 c) Severe burns
 d) Iron deficiency
 e) Obstructive jaundice

35. Which of the following are hepatotoxic?

 a) Dextropropoxyphene
 b) Di-isocyanates
 c) Polyvinylchloride
 d) Pyrazinamide
 e) Dioxine

36. In hypokalaemia the following occur:

    a) T waves on the ECG increase in size
    b) ST segment depression occurs
    c) U waves appear
    d) The QT interval is shortened
    e) The QRS complex widens

37. Metronidazole is effective against:

    a) *Bacteroides*
    b) *Trichomonas vaginalis*
    c) *Entamoeba histolytica*
    d) *Taenia solium*
    e) *Diphyllobothrium latum*

38. Which of these drugs are best avoided in pregnancy?

    a) Digoxin
    b) Carbimazole
    c) Chloramphenicol
    d) Phenytoin
    e) Warfarin

39. Hypoglycaemia may:

    a) Result from chlorpropamide therapy
    b) Herald the onset of diabetes mellitus
    c) Cause prolonged cerebral dysfunction
    d) Be reversed by glucagon
    e) Occur in the Zollinger-Ellison syndrome

40. Gynaecomastia may result from:

    a) Sarcoidosis
    b) Carcinoma of the bronchus
    c) Hypertrichosis lanuginosa
    d) Prednisone therapy
    e) Cimetidine therapy

41. Red scaling skin lesions are seen in:

   a) Urticaria
   b) Tinea cruris
   c) Secondary syphilis
   d) Pityriasis versicolor
   e) Dermatitis herpetiformis

42. Which of these haemodynamic pressures are normal?

   a) Left atrium 10 mmHg
   b) Left ventricle 125/8 mmHg
   c) Aorta 190/40 mmHg
   d) Pulmonary artery 60/30 mmHg
   e) Right atrium 35 mmHg

43. Which of these statements are true in right ventricular failure?

   a) Pulmonary artery wedge pressure is unaffected
   b) Emphysema is a rare cause
   c) Pulsus alternans occurs
   d) Left ventricular ejection fraction is usually reduced
   e) Central venous pressure is usually greater than 4 mmHg

44. Hypokalaemia may result from:

   a) Anorexia nervosa
   b) Ulcerative colitis
   c) Purgative abuse
   d) Coeliac disease
   e) Diabetes mellitus

45. Which names are most associated with aortic incompetence?

   a) Graham Steell
   b) Durozier
   c) Corrigan
   d) Quincke
   e) Marfan

46. Specific heart muscle disease may result from:

   a) Vitamin B_1 deficiency
   b) Cholera
   c) Cushing's syndrome
   d) Carcinoid syndrome
   e) Scleroderma

47. The following pulmonary infections are diagnostic of AIDS in a high-risk patient:

   a) *Mycobacterium tuberculosis*
   b) Cytomegalovirus pneumonia
   c) *Legionella pneumophila*
   d) *Pneumocystis carinii* pneumonia
   'e) Lung abscess due to *Streptococcus milleri*

48. Which of these statements are true of lymphogranuloma venereum?

   a) It is due to infection with *Chlamydia* species
   b) It is common in tropical climates
   c) The primary lesion is a painful nodule
   d) Elephantiasis may occur
   e) Painless lymphadenopathy is usual

49. Which of the following are causes of generalised lymphadenopathy?

   a) EB virus
   b) Syphilis
   c) HTLV-III
   d) *Toxoplasma gondii*
   e) Q fever

50. Rabies:

   a) Is spread by cats as well as dogs
   b) Is common in California
   c) May be associated with fasciculation near the bite
   d) Causes aerophobia
   e) Often causes papilloedema

51. The right vertebral artery:

a) Is a branch of the aorta
b) Traverses the foramina of the upper five cervical vertebrae
c) Meets the left vertebral artery to form the basilar artery
d) Crosses the dome of the pleura
e) Runs on the postero-lateral aspect of the medulla

52. A IVth cranial nerve palsy:

a) Involves loss of depression of the eye in the abducted position
b) When bilateral, is usually secondary to trauma
c) Shows defective torsion of the eye
d) Is associated with a dilated pupil on the side of the lesion
e) Can be due to cavernous sinus infection

53. Acetylator status is clinically important with which of the following drug therapies?

a) Propranolol
b) Hydralazine
c) Dapsone
d) Penicillin
e) Isoniazid

54. Griseofulvin is an effective treatment of infection with:

a) *Candida albicans*
b) *Trichophyton rubra*
c) *Microsporum canis*
d) *Malassezia furfur*
e) *Taenia solium*

55. Which of the following are alpha sympathetic effects?

a) Uterine relaxation
b) Vasoconstriction
c) Relaxation of the radial muscle of the iris
d) Gut relaxation
e) Bronchial relaxation

56. A purpuric rash may occur in:

a) Typhus
b) Gonorrhoea
c) Yellow fever
d) Congenital cytomegalovirus infection
e) Acquired rubella

57. Which of the following are usually indications for cardiac artificial pacemakers?

a) Trifascicular block
b) First degree AV block
c) Second degree AV block — Mobitz type I
d) Sinoatrial disease
e) Acquired third degree nodal block

58. Which is statistically significant?

a) $r = -1$
b) $P \leqslant 0.5$
c) $t = 1$
d) $P \leqslant 0.01$
e) $x^2 = 0.5$

59. Antidiuretic hormone (ADH):

a) Is a short peptide
b) Is synthesised in the infraoptic and proventricular nuclei of the hypothalamus
c) Travels by axonal streaming
d) Acts on the distal renal tubule
e) Has a plasma half-life of about 60 min

60. Which of the following disorders are usually of T cell origin?

a) Burkitt's lymphoma
b) Hodgkin's disease
c) Chronic lymphocytic leukaemia
d) Mycosis fungoides
e) Sezary's syndrome

Examinations

Examination 5

All parts of every Question
must be answered *True* or *False*
or *Don't Know* by filling in the
box provided. Failure to do so
will result in rejection of the
answer sheet

EXAMINATION NO.
5

SURNAME

INITIALS

Please use 2B PENCIL only. Rub out all errors thoroughly.
Mark lozenges like ▬ <u>NOT</u> like this ⊄ ⊄ ⊗

T ⬭ = TRUE   F ⬭ = FALSE   DK ⬭ = DON'T KNOW

	A	B	C	D	E
1	T ⬭ F ⬭ DK ⬭	T ⬭ F ⬭ DK ⬭	T ⬭ F ⬭ DK ⬭	T ⬭ F ⬭ DK ⬭	T ⬭ F ⬭ DK ⬭
2	T ⬭ F ⬭ DK ⬭	T ⬭ F ⬭ DK ⬭	T ⬭ F ⬭ DK ⬭	T ⬭ F ⬭ DK ⬭	T ⬭ F ⬭ DK ⬭
3	T ⬭ F ⬭ DK ⬭	T ⬭ F ⬭ DK ⬭	T ⬭ F ⬭ DK ⬭	T ⬭ F ⬭ DK ⬭	T ⬭ F ⬭ DK ⬭
4	T ⬭ F ⬭ DK ⬭	T ⬭ F ⬭ DK ⬭	T ⬭ F ⬭ DK ⬭	T ⬭ F ⬭ DK ⬭	T ⬭ F ⬭ DK ⬭
5	T ⬭ F ⬭ DK ⬭	T ⬭ F ⬭ DK ⬭	T ⬭ F ⬭ DK ⬭	T ⬭ F ⬭ DK ⬭	T ⬭ F ⬭ DK ⬭
6	T ⬭ F ⬭ DK ⬭	T ⬭ F ⬭ DK ⬭	T ⬭ F ⬭ DK ⬭	T ⬭ F ⬭ DK ⬭	T ⬭ F ⬭ DK ⬭
7	T ⬭ F ⬭ DK ⬭	T ⬭ F ⬭ DK ⬭	T ⬭ F ⬭ DK ⬭	T ⬭ F ⬭ DK ⬭	T ⬭ F ⬭ DK ⬭
8	T ⬭ F ⬭ DK ⬭	T ⬭ F ⬭ DK ⬭	T ⬭ F ⬭ DK ⬭	T ⬭ F ⬭ DK ⬭	T ⬭ F ⬭ DK ⬭
9	T ⬭ F ⬭ DK ⬭	T ⬭ F ⬭ DK ⬭	T ⬭ F ⬭ DK ⬭	T ⬭ F ⬭ DK ⬭	T ⬭ F ⬭ DK ⬭
10	T ⬭ F ⬭ DK ⬭	T ⬭ F ⬭ DK ⬭	T ⬭ F ⬭ DK ⬭	T ⬭ F ⬭ DK ⬭	T ⬭ F ⬭ DK ⬭
11	T ⬭ F ⬭ DK ⬭	T ⬭ F ⬭ DK ⬭	T ⬭ F ⬭ DK ⬭	T ⬭ F ⬭ DK ⬭	T ⬭ F ⬭ DK ⬭
12	T ⬭ F ⬭ DK ⬭	T ⬭ F ⬭ DK ⬭	T ⬭ F ⬭ DK ⬭	T ⬭ F ⬭ DK ⬭	T ⬭ F ⬭ DK ⬭
13	T ⬭ F ⬭ DK ⬭	T ⬭ F ⬭ DK ⬭	T ⬭ F ⬭ DK ⬭	T ⬭ F ⬭ DK ⬭	T ⬭ F ⬭ DK ⬭
14	T ⬭ F ⬭ DK ⬭	T ⬭ F ⬭ DK ⬭	T ⬭ F ⬭ DK ⬭	T ⬭ F ⬭ DK ⬭	T ⬭ F ⬭ DK ⬭
15	T ⬭ F ⬭ DK ⬭	T ⬭ F ⬭ DK ⬭	T ⬭ F ⬭ DK ⬭	T ⬭ F ⬭ DK ⬭	T ⬭ F ⬭ DK ⬭

	A	B	C	D	E
16	T ⬭ F ⬭ DK ⬭	T ⬭ F ⬭ DK ⬭	T ⬭ F ⬭ DK ⬭	T ⬭ F ⬭ DK ⬭	T ⬭ F ⬭ DK ⬭
17	T ⬭ F ⬭ DK ⬭	T ⬭ F ⬭ DK ⬭	T ⬭ F ⬭ DK ⬭	T ⬭ F ⬭ DK ⬭	T ⬭ F ⬭ DK ⬭
18	T ⬭ F ⬭ DK ⬭	T ⬭ F ⬭ DK ⬭	T ⬭ F ⬭ DK ⬭	T ⬭ F ⬭ DK ⬭	T ⬭ F ⬭ DK ⬭
19	T ⬭ F ⬭ DK ⬭	T ⬭ F ⬭ DK ⬭	T ⬭ F ⬭ DK ⬭	T ⬭ F ⬭ DK ⬭	T ⬭ F ⬭ DK ⬭
20	T ⬭ F ⬭ DK ⬭	T ⬭ F ⬭ DK ⬭	T ⬭ F ⬭ DK ⬭	T ⬭ F ⬭ DK ⬭	T ⬭ F ⬭ DK ⬭
21	T ⬭ F ⬭ DK ⬭	T ⬭ F ⬭ DK ⬭	T ⬭ F ⬭ DK ⬭	T ⬭ F ⬭ DK ⬭	T ⬭ F ⬭ DK ⬭
22	T ⬭ F ⬭ DK ⬭	T ⬭ F ⬭ DK ⬭	T ⬭ F ⬭ DK ⬭	T ⬭ F ⬭ DK ⬭	T ⬭ F ⬭ DK ⬭
23	T ⬭ F ⬭ DK ⬭	T ⬭ F ⬭ DK ⬭	T ⬭ F ⬭ DK ⬭	T ⬭ F ⬭ DK ⬭	T ⬭ F ⬭ DK ⬭
24	T ⬭ F ⬭ DK ⬭	T ⬭ F ⬭ DK ⬭	T ⬭ F ⬭ DK ⬭	T ⬭ F ⬭ DK ⬭	T ⬭ F ⬭ DK ⬭
25	T ⬭ F ⬭ DK ⬭	T ⬭ F ⬭ DK ⬭	T ⬭ F ⬭ DK ⬭	T ⬭ F ⬭ DK ⬭	T ⬭ F ⬭ DK ⬭
26	T ⬭ F ⬭ DK ⬭	T ⬭ F ⬭ DK ⬭	T ⬭ F ⬭ DK ⬭	T ⬭ F ⬭ DK ⬭	T ⬭ F ⬭ DK ⬭
27	T ⬭ F ⬭ DK ⬭	T ⬭ F ⬭ DK ⬭	T ⬭ F ⬭ DK ⬭	T ⬭ F ⬭ DK ⬭	T ⬭ F ⬭ DK ⬭
28	T ⬭ F ⬭ DK ⬭	T ⬭ F ⬭ DK ⬭	T ⬭ F ⬭ DK ⬭	T ⬭ F ⬭ DK ⬭	T ⬭ F ⬭ DK ⬭
29	T ⬭ F ⬭ DK ⬭	T ⬭ F ⬭ DK ⬭	T ⬭ F ⬭ DK ⬭	T ⬭ F ⬭ DK ⬭	T ⬭ F ⬭ DK ⬭
30	T ⬭ F ⬭ DK ⬭	T ⬭ F ⬭ DK ⬭	T ⬭ F ⬭ DK ⬭	T ⬭ F ⬭ DK ⬭	T ⬭ F ⬭ DK ⬭

	A	B	C	D	E		A	B	C	D	E
31	T ○ F ○ DK ○	T ○ F ○ DK ○	T ○ F ○ DK ○	T ○ F ○ DK ○	T ○ F ○ DK ○	**46**	T ○ F ○ DK ○	T ○ F ○ DK ○	T ○ F ○ DK ○	T ○ F ○ DK ○	T ○ F ○ DK ○
32	T ○ F ○ DK ○	T ○ F ○ DK ○	T ○ F ○ DK ○	T ○ F ○ DK ○	T ○ F ○ DK ○	**47**	T ○ F ○ DK ○	T ○ F ○ DK ○	T ○ F ○ DK ○	T ○ F ○ DK ○	T ○ F ○ DK ○
33	T ○ F ○ DK ○	T ○ F ○ DK ○	T ○ F ○ DK ○	T ○ F ○ DK ○	T ○ F ○ DK ○	**48**	T ○ F ○ DK ○	T ○ F ○ DK ○	T ○ F ○ DK ○	T ○ F ○ DK ○	T ○ F ○ DK ○
34	T ○ F ○ DK ○	T ○ F ○ DK ○	T ○ F ○ DK ○	T ○ F ○ DK ○	T ○ F ○ DK ○	**49**	T ○ F ○ DK ○	T ○ F ○ DK ○	T ○ F ○ DK ○	T ○ F ○ DK ○	T ○ F ○ DK ○
35	T ○ F ○ DK ○	T ○ F ○ DK ○	T ○ F ○ DK ○	T ○ F ○ DK ○	T ○ F ○ DK ○	**50**	T ○ F ○ DK ○	T ○ F ○ DK ○	T ○ F ○ DK ○	T ○ F ○ DK ○	T ○ F ○ DK ○
36	T ○ F ○ DK ○	T ○ F ○ DK ○	T ○ F ○ DK ○	T ○ F ○ DK ○	T ○ F ○ DK ○	**51**	T ○ F ○ DK ○	T ○ F ○ DK ○	T ○ F ○ DK ○	T ○ F ○ DK ○	T ○ F ○ DK ○
37	T ○ F ○ DK ○	T ○ F ○ DK ○	T ○ F ○ DK ○	T ○ F ○ DK ○	T ○ F ○ DK ○	**52**	T ○ F ○ DK ○	T ○ F ○ DK ○	T ○ F ○ DK ○	T ○ F ○ DK ○	T ○ F ○ DK ○
38	T ○ F ○ DK ○	T ○ F ○ DK ○	T ○ F ○ DK ○	T ○ F ○ DK ○	T ○ F ○ DK ○	**53**	T ○ F ○ DK ○	T ○ F ○ DK ○	T ○ F ○ DK ○	T ○ F ○ DK ○	T ○ F ○ DK ○
39	T ○ F ○ DK ○	T ○ F ○ DK ○	T ○ F ○ DK ○	T ○ F ○ DK ○	T ○ F ○ DK ○	**54**	T ○ F ○ DK ○	T ○ F ○ DK ○	T ○ F ○ DK ○	T ○ F ○ DK ○	T ○ F ○ DK ○
40	T ○ F ○ DK ○	T ○ F ○ DK ○	T ○ F ○ DK ○	T ○ F ○ DK ○	T ○ F ○ DK ○	**55**	T ○ F ○ DK ○	T ○ F ○ DK ○	T ○ F ○ DK ○	T ○ F ○ DK ○	T ○ F ○ DK ○
41	T ○ F ○ DK ○	T ○ F ○ DK ○	T ○ F ○ DK ○	T ○ F ○ DK ○	T ○ F ○ DK ○	**56**	T ○ F ○ DK ○	T ○ F ○ DK ○	T ○ F ○ DK ○	T ○ F ○ DK ○	T ○ F ○ DK ○
42	T ○ F ○ DK ○	T ○ F ○ DK ○	T ○ F ○ DK ○	T ○ F ○ DK ○	T ○ F ○ DK ○	**57**	T ○ F ○ DK ○	T ○ F ○ DK ○	T ○ F ○ DK ○	T ○ F ○ DK ○	T ○ F ○ DK ○
43	T ○ F ○ DK ○	T ○ F ○ DK ○	T ○ F ○ DK ○	T ○ F ○ DK ○	T ○ F ○ DK ○	**58**	T ○ F ○ DK ○	T ○ F ○ DK ○	T ○ F ○ DK ○	T ○ F ○ DK ○	T ○ F ○ DK ○
44	T ○ F ○ DK ○	T ○ F ○ DK ○	T ○ F ○ DK ○	T ○ F ○ DK ○	T ○ F ○ DK ○	**59**	T ○ F ○ DK ○	T ○ F ○ DK ○	T ○ F ○ DK ○	T ○ F ○ DK ○	T ○ F ○ DK ○
45	T ○ F ○ DK ○	T ○ F ○ DK ○	T ○ F ○ DK ○	T ○ F ○ DK ○	T ○ F ○ DK ○	**60**	T ○ F ○ DK ○	T ○ F ○ DK ○	T ○ F ○ DK ○	T ○ F ○ DK ○	T ○ F ○ DK ○

1. Which drugs induce hepatic microsomal enzymes?

   a) Rifampicin
   b) Lorazepam
   c) Phenytoin
   d) Trimethoprim
   e) Paracetamol

2. Which of the following diseases affect the retina?

   a) Tay Sachs disease
   b) Pseudoxanthoma elasticum
   c) *Toxocara canis* infection
   d) Bronchiectasis
   e) Heterochromic cyclitis

3. The sciatic nerve:

   a) Is formed from L4, 5, S1, 2, 3 nerve roots
   b) Emerges from the lesser sciatic foramen
   c) Is crossed by the long head of the biceps femoris
   d) Divides into the tibial and common peroneal nerves
   e) Branches supply vastus medialis

4. A litre of human milk compared with a litre of cow's milk contains more:

   a) Fat
   b) Sodium
   c) Vitamin C
   d) Calories
   e) Chloride

5. Common pathogens in neonates are:

   a) *Escherichia coli*
   b) *Listeria monocytogenes*
   c) *Streptococcus pneumoniae*
   d) *Cryptosporidiosis*
   e) *Giardia lamblia*

6. Which of the following drugs (taken in usual dosages) may have psychiatric side-effects?

   a) Benzhexol
   b) Ibuprofen
   c) Digitalis
   d) Isoniazid
   e) Rifampicin

7. Psychiatric disorders related to alcohol include:

   a) Short-term amnesia
   b) Suicidal behaviour
   c) Psychosexual dysfunction
   d) Pathological jealousy
   e) Auditory hallucinations

8. In cannabis smokers:

   a) A withdrawal syndrome is common
   b) Tolerance occurs
   c) Cerebral atrophy may occur
   d) Psychosis commonly occurs
   e) Increased salivation occurs

9. The following often occur after small intestinal resection:

   a) Gastric hypersecretion
   b) Cathartic diarrhoea
   c) Uric acid renal stones
   d) Cholesterol gallstones
   e) An abnormal glycocholate C^{14} breath test

10. In acute viral hepatitis:

    a) Bed rest protects patients against a more severe illness
    b) Fat in the diet impairs recovery
    c) Clinical relapse is commoner if treated with corticosteroids
    d) A high protein diet is contraindicated because of the risk of precipitating encephalopathy
    e) A low blood sugar is often found

11. Complications of ulcerative colitis include:

    a) Venous thrombosis
    b) Arterial thrombosis
    c) Episcleritis
    d) Aphthous ulcers
    e) Infertility in women

12. In the normal pancreas:

    a) Glucagon is produced from gamma cells
    b) Digestive enzymes are produced from acinar cells
    c) Proteolytic enzymes are activated in the duodenum
    d) Water and electrolytes are secreted in response to secretin
    e) Pancreatic secretion is inhibited by vagally mediated reflexes

13. Renal artery stenosis is demonstrated on an intravenous urogram by:

    a) Early appearance of contrast on the affected side
    b) Increased density of contrast on late films on the affected side
    c) A smaller kidney on the affected side
    d) High volume collecting systems
    e) Late filling of the renal veins

14. Which of the following can cause interstitial nephritis?

    a) Leprosy
    b) Hodgkin's disease
    c) Renal vein thrombosis
    d) Familial Mediterranean fever
    e) Uric acid nephropathy

15. Problems associated with regular haemodialysis include:

    a) Cramps
    b) Dementia
    c) Impotence
    d) Myocardial infarction
    e) Ruptured muscle tendons

16. Concerning folate metabolism, which statements are true?
    a) Folate is required in the synthesis of thymidine monophosphate
    b) B_{12} is needed in the conversion of tetrahydrofolate to methyl- tetrahydrofolate
    c) All dietary folate is converted to methyl-tetrahydrofolate
    d) Bacterial folate synthesis is inhibited by sulphonamides
    e) The enzyme dihydrofolate reductase is induced by pyrimethamine

17. In diabetic renal disease:
    a) Insulin needs decrease by up to 50% in established renal failure
    b) Focal nodular sclerosis is the usual histological finding
    c) Basement membrane thickening is the earliest histological feature
    d) The glomerular filtration rate is increased in early renal disease
    e) Nephrotic syndrome will resolve with good diabetic control

18. Which are true of a normal distribution?
    a) 60% of observations are within one standard deviation of the mean
    b) The standard error is greater than the standard deviation
    c) The distribution has a bell-shaped curve
    d) 95% of observations fall within two standard deviations of the mean
    e) It is also normally distributed if converted to a log/log plot

19. In kernicterus:
    a) The bilirubin is rarely over 250 μmol/litre
    b) Intelligence is classically preserved
    c) Blindness is common
    d) There may be paralysis of upward gaze
    e) The Crigler-Najjar syndrome does not have the same neurological sequelae

20. Which of the following conditions are inherited in an autosomal dominant form?
    a) Cystic fibrosis
    b) Homocystinuria
    c) Von Willebrand's syndrome
    d) Achondroplasia
    e) Tuberous sclerosis

21. Hyperventilation may result from:

    a) Marathon running
    b) Pneumothorax
    c) The 'bends'
    d) Tetanus
    e) Botulism

22. Concerning carbon dioxide, in a normal subject, which of these statements are true?

    a) A rise in $PaCO_2$ causes an increase in respiratory rate
    b) Increase in $PaCO_2$ shifts the oxygen dissociation curve to the left
    c) Carbon dioxide excretion is the main acid–base regulator in the body
    d) Carbon dioxide is a vasodilator
    e) Apnoea may follow a drop in $PaCO_2$

23. Periods of apnoea may occur in:

    a) REM sleep
    b) Healthy subjects at altitude
    c) Cardiac failure
    d) Heroin overdose
    e) Asthma

24. The FEV_1 is characteristically reduced in:

    a) Emphysema
    b) Asthma
    c) Stage I sarcoidosis
    d) Chronic bronchiectasis
    e) Cryptogenic fibrosing alveolitis

25. The ulnar nerve supplies:

    a) Biceps
    b) Medial lumbricals
    c) Flexor carpi ulnaris
    d) Opponens pollicis
    e) Flexor pollicis longus

26. Which of the following may cause cataracts?

    a) Glaucoma
    b) Trauma
    c) Ophthalmitis
    d) Steroid therapy
    e) Intrauterine rubella

27. Papilloedema may result from:

    a) Meningioma
    b) Steroid therapy
    c) Thyrotoxicosis
    d) Type II respiratory failure
    e) Central retinal artery embolus

28. Concerning cerebrovascular accidents, which are true?

    a) Cerebral haemorrhage is rarely fatal
    b) It is essential to keep the diastolic blood pressure below 90 mmHg
    c) The level of consciousness on admission affects prognosis
    d) Headache is diagnostic for cerebral embolism
    e) Recovery is complete by 4 weeks

29. Chylomicrons:

    a) Disappear from the circulation by 4 h after a fatty meal
    b) Are synthesised in the liver
    c) Are increased in type IIa hyperlipidaemia
    d) Float to the surface of normal samples
    e) In excess, are associated with pancreatitis

30. Hyponatraemia may occur in:

    a) Heavy beer drinkers
    b) Cushing's disease
    c) Hypothyroidism
    d) Diabetes insipidus
    e) Treatment with metolazone

31. Which of the following may occur as a result of treatment for rheumatoid arthritis?

    a) Myasthenia gravis
    b) Nephrotic syndrome
    c) Blindness
    d) Corneal deposits
    e) Goodpasture's syndrome

32. Felty's syndrome is characterised by:

    a) Hepatomegaly
    b) Pulmonary nodules
    c) Panniculitis
    d) Leucopenia
    e) Pericarditis

33. Sacro-iliac joints are often affected in:

    a) Rheumatoid arthritis
    b) Serum sickness
    c) Psoriatic arthropathy
    d) Brucellosis
    e) Reiter's syndrome

34. Bowing of the tibia occurs in:

    a) Scurvy
    b) Osteoporosis
    c) Paget's disease
    d) Syphilis
    e) Adult Fanconi syndrome

35. Which of the following are markers for, or dependent upon, B-lymphocytes?

    a) PHA response
    b) C3 receptors
    c) Lipopolysaccharide (LPS) response
    d) PPD response
    e) Sheep red blood cell rosette formation

36. Sideroblastic anaemia may result from:

    a) Disseminated malignancy
    b) Carbon monoxide poisoning
    c) Lead poisoning
    d) Ethambutol therapy
    e) Uraemia

37. With respect to the oxyhaemoglobin dissociation curve, which are true? There is:

    a) A shift to the right with anaemia
    b) A shift to the left with increases in 2,3-diphosphoglycerate
    c) A shift to the right with a rise in pH
    d) A shift to the left with a rise in temperature
    e) No shift with a rise in carboxyhaemoglobin

38. Which of the following are recognised features of alpha-1-antitrypsin deficiency?

    a) Sex-linked inheritance
    b) Cirrhosis of the liver
    c) Pancreatitis
    d) Hypospadias
    e) Recurrent pulmonary infections

39. Raynaud's syndrome may be helped by:

    a) Prostacyclin
    b) Nifedipine
    c) Propranolol
    d) Cinnarizine
    e) Dobutamine

40. Which of these drugs should only be used with caution in renal failure?

    a) Cimetidine
    b) Isoniazid
    c) Aspirin
    d) Tobramycin
    e) Atenolol

41. Complications of treatment with rifampicin are:

   a) Contraceptive pill failure
   b) Renal tubular necrosis
   c) Peripheral neuropathy
   d) Suicide
   e) Hepatitis

42. Amenorrhoea may result from:

   a) Bulimia
   b) Arrhenoblastoma
   c) Pulmonary tuberculosis
   d) Adrenogenital syndrome
   e) Alcoholism

43. Which of the following factors cause increased renin secretion?

   a) Cortisol
   b) Standing up
   c) Hypertension
   d) Angiotensin II
   e) Treatment with thiazide diuretics

44. Onycholysis is seen in:

   a) Thyroid acropachy
   b) Acromegaly
   c) Candidal paronychia
   d) Psoriasis
   e) Clubbing due to cyanotic congenital heart disease

45. In coronary angiography, which are true?

   a) Catheterisation of the left coronary artery is safer than that of the right
   b) Cerebral embolism may occur
   c) Mortality is under 0.5%
   d) The radial pulse may be absent afterwards
   e) Prophylactic heparin reduces morbidity

46. The PR interval on the ECG is increased in:

a) Wolff-Parkinson-White syndrome
b) Sino-atrial block
c) Bifascicular block
d) Mobitz type II block
e) Wenckebach phenomenon

47. Which of these associations in jugular venous waveform are found?

a) Cannon waves — multiple ventricular extrasystoles
b) Fast y descent — triscupid stenosis
c) Absent a waves — atrial flutter
d) Large v waves — constrictive pericarditis
e) Giant a wave — tricuspid incompetence

48. Subacute bacterial endocarditis may occur with which of the following?

a) Ventricular aneurysm
b) Ventricular septal defect
c) Hypertrophic obstructive cardiomyopathy
d) Normal heart valves
e) Tricuspid atresia

49. Pericarditis may result from:

a) Myxoedema
b) Beri-Beri
c) Tuberculosis
d) Rheumatic fever
e) Systemic lupus erythematosus

50. Brucellosis:

a) Is carried by snails
b) Causes a leucocytosis
c) Is common in cows in the United Kingdom
d) Causes a relative tachycardia
e) May be diagnosed by bone marrow culture

51. Rubella in the early weeks of intrauterine life may cause:

   a) Cleft palate
   b) Cardiac abnormalities
   c) Spina bifida
   d) Deafness
   e) Cataracts

52. Which of the following exert their effects by exotoxins?

   a) Beta streptococcus
   b) Gonorrhoea
   c) *Staphylococcus aureus*
   d) *Shigella dysenteriae*
   e) *Salmonella* spp.

53. Human T cell lymphotropic virus III (HTLV-III) is:

   a) Only found in homosexuals
   b) A retrovirus
   c) A cause of generalised lymphadenopathy
   d) Cytotoxic for B cells
   e) A lung pathogen

54. Bacteriostatic drugs include:

   a) Rifampicin
   b) Chloramphenicol
   c) Gentamicin
   d) Co-trimoxazole
   e) Erythromycin

55. The following drugs undergo first pass metabolism in the liver:

   a) Propranolol
   b) Lignocaine
   c) Testosterone
   d) Stilboestrol
   e) Nortriptyline

56. Vesicles occur in which of these diseases?

   a) Herpangina
   b) Behçet's disease
   c) Trichinosis
   d) Molluscum contagiosum
   e) Dengue fever

57. Giant a waves may commonly be seen in the jugular venous pulse with:

   a) Mitral valvotomy
   b) An artificial ventricular pacemaker
   c) Ventricular tachycardia
   d) Atrial ectopics
   e) Tricuspid incompetence

58. The serum phosphate:

   a) Is normal in hypoparathyroidism
   b) Is low in rickets
   c) Is high in pseudopseudohypoparathyroidism
   d) Is normal in pseudohypoparathyroidism
   e) Is low in senile osteoporosis

59. Which of the following vaccinations are live attentuated viruses?

   a) Influenza
   b) BCG
   c) Rabies
   d) Rubella
   e) Yellow fever

60. Which of the following may cause a hyperchloraemic acidosis?

   a) Pyloric stenosis
   b) Acetozolamide therapy
   c) Ingestion of vitamin C in high dosage
   d) Ureterosigmoid anastomosis
   e) A 24-hour sodium intake of 250 mmol

Answers

Examination 1
(Pass mark 130/300)

1. True — a, b, d
2. True — d
3. True — b
4. True — none
5. True — b, c
6. True — b, e
7. True — c, d
8. True — a, d
9. True — b, d
10. True — c
11. True — a, c
12. True — c, d
13. True — a, c
14. True — a, c, d
15. True — c, d
16. True — b, e
17. True — a, b, e
18. True — a, b, c, e
19. True — a, c, d, e
20. True — a, d, e
21. True — c, e
22. True — b, c
23. True — a, c, d
24. True — b
25. True — c, e
26. True — b, c, d
27. True — a, b
28. True — a, b, c
29. True — a, d
30. True — d, e

31. True — a, b, e
32. True — a, c, d, e
33. True — a, d
34. True — b, c
35. True — a, c
36. True — a
37. True — b
38. True — a, d, e
39. True — d
40. True — a, b, c, d, e
41. True — a
42. True — c, d
43. True — c, d
44. True — a, b
45. True — c, d, e
46. True — c
47. True — a, b, d
48. True — b, e
49. True — a, b, d
50. True — a, b, c, d, e
51. True — a, b, d, e
52. True — a, b, d
53. True — a, b, c, d, e
54. True — a, e
55. True — c, e
56. True — c, e
57. True — b, e
58. True — a, b, c, d
59. True — b, d, e
60. True — a, b, c, d, e

Examination 2
(Pass mark 150/300)

1. True — a, b, c, e
2. True — a, b, d, e
3. True — a, c, d
4. True — d
5. True — d, e
6. True — c, e
7. True — a, c, d
8. True — a, b, c, e
9. True — a, b, e
10. True — a, b, c
11. True — a, b, d
12. True — a, e
13. True — c, e
14. True — d, e
15. True — a, b, d
16. True — a, d, e
17. True — a, c
18. True — a, b, e
19. True — c, e
20. True — a, b, c
21. True — b, e
22. True — a, c
23. True — b, e
24. True — a, b, e
25. True — b, d, e
26. True — a, b, d, e
27. True — a
28. True — a, c
29. True — a, b, c, d, e
30. True — a, b, e

31. True — a, b, d, e
32. True — b, c, d
33. True — b, c
34. True — b, c, d
35. True — c, d, e
36. True — a, b, d
37. True — e
38. True — b, e
39. True — a, b, d
40. True — e
41. True — c, d, e
42. True — a, e
43. True — none
44. True — a, c, e
45. True — a, d
46. True — b, d
47. True — a, b, c, d
48. True — a, b, d, e
49. True — a, b, c, d, e
50. True — b, c, e
51. True — a, c
52. True — b, d
53. True — b, c, d
54. True — b, c
55. True — c, d, e
56. True — none
57. True — c
58. True — c, d, e
59. True — b, e
60. True — b, c

Examination 3
(Pass mark 165/300)

1. True — b, d, e
2. True — a, c, d, e
3. True — a, b, d, e
4. True — a, b, d
5. True — a, c, d
6. True — a, b, c, d
7. True — b, d, e
8. True — a, b, c
9. True — a, b
10. True — c
11. True — a, b, c
12. True — a, b, c, d
13. True — a, c, d
14. True — c, d
15. True — b, d
16. True — b, d, e
17. True — c, d, e
18. True — c, d
19. True — a, b, d
20. True — a, b, c, d
21. True — a
22. True — a, b, c
23. True — d
24. True — a, b, c, e
25. True — a
26. True — b, d
27. True — b
28. True — b, d, e
29. True — c, e
30. True — b, d

31. True — a, b, d, e
32. True — a, c, e
33. True — a, b, c, d, e
34. True — b, c
35. True — c, d
36. True — b
37. True — a, b, c
38. True — b, d
39. True — a, b, c, e
40. True — b, d, e
41. True — b, c
42. True — b, c, d
43. True — a, b, c, d
44. True — b, c, e
45. True — a
46. True — b, c, d
47. True — c, d, e
48. True — b, d, e
49. True — b, c, d
50. True — a, b, c
51. True — a, c, e
52. True — b, e
53. True — c, d
54. True — b
55. True — a, c, d
56. True — a, c, d, e
57. True — a, d, e
58. True — a, c, e
59. True — b, d
60. True — b, c, d

Examination 4
(Pass mark 160/300)

1. True — a, b, c, e
2. True — a, d
3. True — a, b, e
4. True — a, b, c
5. True — a, b, c, d
6. True — a, b, d, e
7. True — a, c
8. True — a, c
9. True — a, b, c, d
10. True — b, c, d
11. True — a, c, d
12. True — none
13. True — a, b, c, d, e
14. True — e
15. True — b, d
16. True — c, d
17. True — d, e
18. True — b, d, e
19. True — d, e
20. True — a, b, d
21. True — a
22. True — a, c, d
23. True — c, d, e
24. True — b, d
25. True — a, b, c, d, e
26. True — a, b, c, d, e
27. True — b, c, d, e
28. True — b, d, e
29. True — b, e
30. True — a, b, c, d, e

31. True — a, c, d
32. True — a, c, d
33. True — a, b, c, d, e
34. True — a, b, d, e
35. True — c, d, e
36. True — b, c, e
37. True — a, b, c
38. True — b, c, d, e
39. True — a, b, c, d, e
40. True — b, e
41. True — b, c
42. True — b
43. True — b, c, e
44. True — a, b, c, d, e
45. True — b, c, d, e
46. True — a, e
47. True — b, d
48. True — a, b, d
49. True — b, c, e
50. True — a, b, c, d
51. True — b, c, d
52. True — a, b, c, e
53. True — b, c, e
54. True — b, c
55. True — b
56. True — a, b, c, d, e
57. True — a, d, e
58. True — b, d, e
59. True — a, b, c, d
60. True — d, e

Examination 5
(Pass mark 135/300)

1. True — a, c
2. True — a, b, d
3. True — a, c, d
4. True — c
5. True — a, b
6. True — a, c, d, e
7. True — a, b, c, d, e
8. True — none
9. True — a, b, d, e
10. True — c
11. True — a, b, c, d
12. True — b, c, d
13. True — b, c
14. True — e
15. True — a, b, c, d, e
16. True — a, c, d
17. True — a, c, d
18. True — c, d
19. True — d
20. True — c, d, e
21. True — b, e
22. True — a, c, d, e
23. True — b, c
24. True — a, b, d, e
25. True — b, c, e
26. True — a, b, c, d, e
27. True — a, b, c, d
28. True — c
29. True — d, e
30. True — a, c, e

31. True — a, b, c, d, e
32. True — d
33. True — c, d, e
34. True — c, d
35. True — b, c, d
36. True — c
37. True — none
38. True — b
39. True — a, b, d
40. True — a, b, c, d, e
41. True — a, e
42. True — a, b, c, d
43. True — b, e
44. True — a, d
45. True — b, c, d, e
46. True — e
47. True — a, c
48. True — b, d, e
49. True — a, c, d, e
50. True — b, e
51. True — b, d, e
52. True — a, c, d
53. True — b, c
54. True — b, e
55. True — a, b, e
56. True — a
57. True — b, c, d
58. True — b
59. True — d, e
60. True — b, d

GPSR Compliance

The European Union's (EU) General Product Safety Regulation (GPSR) is a set of rules that requires consumer products to be safe and our obligations to ensure this.

If you have any concerns about our products, you can contact us on ProductSafety@springernature.com

In case Publisher is established outside the EU, the EU authorized representative is:

Springer Nature Customer Service Center GmbH
Europaplatz 3
69115 Heidelberg, Germany

Batch number: 09635029

Printed by Printforce, the Netherlands